Then, Now and In Between

A Nurse's Story

Mary Curtin Meldazis

Then, Now and In Between
A Nurse's Story
Mary Curtin Meldazis

Cover Design by Pam Feltes of Photography by Feltes
Aurora, Illinois

ISBN-10: 1442134232
ISBN-13: 9781442134232

Printed in the United States of America.

Dedication

This book is dedicated to caregivers worldwide.

Acknowledgements

To my late husband Frank who gave me so much support and encouragement during my career.

My children Matthew, Daniel, and Maura and my son-in-law Frank who are always there for me.

My eight grandchildren of whom I am immensely proud and who keep me young at heart. Thank you to my granddaughter Arielle Penuelas, who portrayed a modern day nurse on the cover.

My family and friends in Ireland, Germany and the United States.

Dr. Donald Nash for his encouragement. He was the sounding board for some of this book and assisted me in choosing the title.

My wonderful friend Caroline Podvin, who helped edit this book and helped compile the glossary. Thank you Caroline for Ro-Jo.

My nursing colleagues too numerous to mention individually. You have made my memories so great.

CHAPTER ONE

This is not an autobiography, but a story of my observations of some of the changes that have occurred in the nursing profession in the past fifty-seven years. It is also a discussion on my experience of the various positions available within the field of nursing.

I grew up in a farming community near the village of Rockchapel in County Cork, Ireland. I was the youngest of four children. I attended the local national school until I was thirteen years old and then attended the Convent of Mercy Secondary (high) School.

I always loved animals and took care of sick or wounded birds and rabbits. I played with the baby calves and piglets and I remember my Dad advising me not to become too attached, as they would eventually be sold.

I cannot recall exactly when I decided I wanted to become a nurse but I remember discussing it with my Mom and asking her where the money would come from for entrance fees. My Mom told me to do well in school and she would find a way. In Ireland, like most of post World War II Europe, times were tough economically.

Though we lived on a farm and always had enough food, money was a scarce commodity. My Mom raised hens and sold the chickens and eggs to a local grocer. She kept the proceeds in the house stored safely in a box. I remember counting it on many occasions. I knew we needed 100 pounds to pay for my entrance fee to the hospital and for uniforms and books. I also needed a watch with a seconds hand to count pulses and respirations. By the time I had completed high school, my Mom had saved enough money. However, there was a waiting list to get into the hospital of my choice.

I began my nursing career as a probationary nurse with on the job training. It was a skin and cancer (S & C) hospital affiliated with the general hospital at which I hoped I would take my nurses training of three years duration.

In the S & C hospital, I learned how to do general house cleaning, simple cooking and bed making. The reason for this work was that I needed to learn to take care of the environment and provide nourishment before I could move on to taking care of a human being.

Bed making was a complicated task and it took me a long time to master the art. All the sheets were flat and the bottom sheet had to be so taut that a big brown penny had to bounce off it. I heard that a quarter was used in the United States.

The corners were envelope corners and the angle had to be just perfect. A half rubber sheet was applied and a draw sheet covered this. These had to cover the bed from approximately the patients' shoulders to the knees. The top sheet, blanket and bedspread were applied separately, all made with envelope corners.

The bedclothes were folded back about twelve inches and the pillow was placed on top. The opening of the pillowcase always faced away from the door. If any part of the bed was incorrectly made, it was pulled apart and I had to start all over again. I spent many hours and shed many tears on bed making.

There were the different types of beds. In a closed bed, the bedclothes were pulled up to enclose the pillow with a pleated effect. If it was an open bed, awaiting the patient's return, the top bedclothes were folded back neatly in thirds.

When a surgical bed was required, the top bedclothes were folded back lengthwise also in thirds. The bed was then ready to receive a patient from a stretcher or cart. Once in bed, the patient could be covered immediately.

At bedtime, the bedspread was removed, folded neatly and placed on a chair, ready for the next day. I often reflect on the need for such precision, but back then, we never wavered from the correct way of doing things.

Now fitted sheets are available and I have encountered floral and printed linens in use. Evidently, the hoopla over bed making is outdated, especially in the healthcare arena.

As I continued in the S & C hospital, I learned the different positions used to assist in caring for patients in various situations.

The recumbent position was laying flat and the semi recumbent position had the head and shoulders a little elevated. The lateral position was side lying either right or left. The prone position had the patient lying on the abdomen with the head turned to either side. The Fowlers position had the upper body at a forty five to sixty degree angle and with the knees bent or straight.

The Fowlers position facilitates breathing and for relaxation of the abdominal muscles after surgery. Charles White, an English physician, first used this position in the early eighteenth century. This position also enables the patient to eat and speak more easily.

A modified version of this is the semi-Fowlers position, where the head is not elevated more than 45°. The next position I learned about was the Trendelenburg position. This involves placing the patient head down with the feet elevated. This position can help counteract shock, by increasing venous return to the heart and improve vital organ perfusion.

My two sons, who are both Eagle Scouts, learned this first aid mnemonic:

> "If the face is red, raise the head and if the face is pale, raise the tail."

It was an American physiologist, Walter Canon, who made this position popular in World War I. Recent research has proven that this theory is a myth but if I had a patient with a low blood pressure or in shock, I would automatically do this. It is often difficult to let go of ideas we have learned so well.

As I progressed in my training, I learned how to give baths, hair, nail care, and transfer patients from a bed to a chair. Patients with various skin conditions, benefited from sulphur baths and the application of tar and sulphur ointments.

During the early 1950s in Ireland, cancer treatments consisted of the use of Radium. Small pieces of Radium, called "seeds" were implanted internally for uterine and rectal cancers. Another treatment consisted of Radium needles with double thick thread inserted through the eye of each needle. The needles were inserted into cancerous skin lesions and into malignant breast tissue. The radiologist determined the length of time the needles would stay in place. I learned how to irrigate the area with a salt-water solution to remove any dead tissue and to count the threads (two threads to one needle in total). Back then, lead aprons were not available to shield staff from radiation.

The use of gloves was very limited at that time. However, our hand washing techniques were beyond reproach. I scrubbed my hands and forearms with a brush, soap and hot water. This was done before and after providing care. After a twelve-hour shift, my arms were often red and sore. Germs were fewer and further between in that time.

As time passed, I learned how to take temperatures, pulses, respiration rates and to test urine for sugar and acetone.

Many changes have occurred in thermometers used to measure body temperature. The first medical thermometer was twelve inches long and took twenty minutes to register. English physician, Sir Thomas Allbutt improved the design to a shorter and faster diagnostic tool that remained nearly unchanged for over a century.

Mercury contained in the glass bulb expands into the glass tube when in contact with body heat. The mercury fluctuates according to temperature and stops at markings along one or both sides of the tube indicating the temperature scale in degrees – Celsius, Fahrenheit or both.

A person's temperature is taken by inserting the tip into the mouth (oral), the rectum (rectal), or the armpit (axillary). The bulb of the oral/axillary thermometer is long, slender and colored blue. The rectal thermometer has a stubbier bulb and is colored red. The color is used to distinguish between thermometer types.

Over the past forty years, the dangers of mercury have been well researched and recognized. Mercury thermometers can be easily broken. The spilled mercury emits a colorless and odorless vapor, which poses health risks if inhaled. Mercury is considered hazardous waste and is expensive to dispose of properly. Many countries have banned the use of mercury thermometers for medical use.

Mercury free thermometers are now in use. Dyed alcohol thermometers are just as accurate and may be used like the mercury ones. Another

non-toxic alternative is the Galistan thermometer, which contains an alloy comprised of gallium,
indium and tin.

In many healthcare settings, electronic thermometers are often used. Sensors inside a
rounded probe can be covered with a disposable
shield to prevent the spread of infection. The
probe is connected to a central processing unit
that collects the temperature reading from the
probe and displays it on an LCD screen. The
probe can be used orally, rectally or axillary.

Once again, technology has produced new methods of measuring body temperature. I have
used an electronic tympanic thermometer that is
used in the ear canal to measure heat from the
eardrum.

Temporal Artery Thermometry utilizes infra-
red technology as a probe is quickly scanned
across the forehead. This accurate and non-
invasive method is very useful for babies and
young children as the temperature can be taken
while they sleep.

CHAPTER TWO

After one year working in the S & C Hospital, I was "called into training" in a general fifty bed hospital. Though my previous training was acknowledged as useful, I was required to start over from scratch.

My uniform consisted of a blue dress with a white collar at the neck, long sleeves with white detachable cuffs, a white apron, black stockings and black shoes. The length of the uniform skirt was mid-calf. When working, we took off the cuffs, rolled up the sleeves and applied a white elastic guard over them.

When allowed out for special church services, I wore a navy blue trench coat and navy blue cap.

I was not allowed to wear a nurse's cap until I had completed three months of general training.

I worked 13 ½ hours every day, seven days a week. The day shift was from 7 a.m. to 8 p.m. beginning and ending with prayer services. I had ½ hour off for breakfast, lunch and supper. I also had a ¼ hour off for afternoon tea.

I received a half day off every other week. I was expected to be in the nurse's dormitory at 8:20 p.m. and it was lights out at 9:30 p.m. I did a lot of my studying with a flashlight hidden under the bedclothes. One night a month, I was allowed out until 11 p.m.

My first three months of training consisted of general housework, washing walls, cleaning toilets and bathtubs, scrubbing floors, polishing brass panels and polishing woodwork. This training was considered essential to prepare someone to care for another human being. My fellow students and I often wondered if it was to save on the housekeeping budget.

After the three months were completed, I took part in a "capping ceremony." I was on my way to becoming a nurse. The next month was spent in the classroom – same hours as working. I learned anatomy, physiology, biology and chemistry. We also practiced bed-making, bathing technique, oral hygiene, vital signs and learned to make general observations. A human skeleton, named Jimmy was available for studying, along with other anatomy and medical charts. When I go into a classroom now and see the learning aids available to students today, I wonder how I ever made it.

My training progressed over a three year period and I was taught medical and surgical nursing, gynecological nursing and male urological nursing. We also studied Pediatrics. In comparison to the present education a Registered Nurse receives, the knowledge was very limited.

When there was a light period in the ward, patients usually napped for 1 to 2 hours after lunch. I rolled pieces of cotton wool into cotton balls, folded laundry, made dressing packs for surgery and sharpened needles for reuse. The syringes were glass, regular 1cc and 5cc and insulin syringes that required sterilization after each use. Dressings were packed in steel drums which were autoclaved and then dated. All autoclaved (sterilized) materials had to be used within three days or they would have to be re-sterilized. Therefore, there was always work to be done in the preparation of needles and dressings.

Nurses working in the operating theatre (surgery) and in the emergency room were responsible for the sterilization of the surgical instruments and dressing packs used in those areas.

During the second and third years of training, I returned to the classroom for another month of study. We were given lectures by the attending physicians and by a sister tutor. Examinations were based on each level of training and the results were posted on the entrance hallways to the wards.

Discipline was strict and it was accepted as a part of my preparation to be a nurse. Each month, a small amount of money was given to each nurse. In the early 1950s, it did not amount to much. We received £3 (about $9). Two shillings and six pence were held back towards an insurance premium.

One day I dropped an insulin syringe and it broke. I had to pay 3 shillings and my monthly privilege of staying out until 11 p.m. was revoked.

On another occasion, the ward sister said I had a bad attitude and my punishment was to fold linen during my lunch break for one week.

Reflecting on those early days of my training, I was often in hot water. One night, I was working on the second floor and had to go down to the first floor to borrow some linen. The hospital did not have elevators, but had two staircases. The front one was made of beautiful highly polished oak with wide banisters and carpeting, used only by the doctors and visitors. The back staircase was made of cement and was for utility purposes and used by everyone else.

As it was the middle of the night and for some other misguided reason, I not only used the front stairway but also slid down the banister. Lo and behold, who was at the bottom but the night sister (the nun in charge)! I was told that I was not a lady and would never make a nurse.

I had to spend an hour in chapel every day for nine days to seek "Divine" guidance. It must have worked because here I am. However, I lost nine hours of sleep and received lots of teasing from my peers, asking why I had become so holy and if I was inspiring to the religious life.

CHAPTER THREE

Care of the sick was through dedicated hard work and a lot of common sense. I honestly believe that God was always close by to direct us with our daily routines. We had a great sense of joy and achievement when a patient got well and went home. The patients spent longer periods in the hospital and we were able to know them better. Visiting hours were limited to two hours on Wednesday and Sunday. If a family lived too far from the hospital, they were unable to visit.

In those days, antibiotics were not available. Surgical patients usually remained in bed between seven to ten days post-op. However, there was always a concern that patients would develop pneumonia or blood clots. To counteract these threats, a patient had to stay in an upright position except during naptime or during sleep at night. Every four hours during the day, from 8 a.m. to 10 p.m. each surgical patient received an inhalation treatment and performed leg exercises.

The inhalation treatment consisted of an earthenware crock filled with boiling water and a tablespoon of an aromatic compound called Friars Balsam.

I have since identified the aroma and in the United States, it is called tincture of Benzoin. We wrapped the crock with a flannel cover to maintain warmth and as a safety measure. The patient was instructed to breathe in the steam through the month and out through the nose for 20 minutes. If the patient was too weak to remain in an upright position for that length of time, the nurse helped support him. I never remember having a patient with respiratory complications following surgery.

Leg exercises consisted of bending and straightening at the hips, knees and ankle joints for a period of ten minutes at least four times a day. This helped to increase circulation and prevent blood clots.

One of the greatest skills that I learned was observation. I was always alert to what may happen. On the medical floors, patients were cared for over a long period. Some were slow to recover from illness.

We did not have intensive care units, so every patient got the utmost care and attention. Patients who survived myocardial infarction (heart attack) stayed on bed rest for 6 weeks.

Nursing care consisted of bathing, skin care, shaving, oral hygiene, repositioning and bed exercises. We did not have electric beds, so Fowlers and Trendelenberg positions were obtained by cranking the head or foot up as needed. If the crank was not returned to its correct position somebody ended up with a bruised shin.

CPR (Cardiopulmonary Resuscitation) was unheard of then, so open cardiac massage was attempted and if the patient survived, the patient became a surgical patient with medical complications.

All the student nurses were young, just out of high school. There were no married nurses back then. People in Ireland married at a later age (late twenties to early thirties). It was assumed a nurse would continue in her profession until she got married. If she entered a religious life or remained single, she could continue in the nursing profession.

In the 1950s, my role as a student nurse was task oriented and dominated by the doctor's orders. On one occasion, I asked a doctor to explain how a sphygmomanometer worked and what did a blood pressure mean. He gruffly told me to stick with TPR's (Temperature, Pulse and Respiration) and I would do OK.

Back then nurses were considered "handmaidens of the doctors", who always stood up when a doctor entered the nurses station and addressed them as Sir. That was then, now we are professionals with our own body of knowledge and are independent thinkers.

Nursing care for patients with medical conditions like rheumatism and arthritis consisted of applications of dry heat in the form of poultices. These were made from scratch, heated in the oven and then applied to the affected limb or joint. There were no microwaves back then. The most common poultices I remember making were made from bran and from a substance called Kaolin. The bran was moistened onto a square of linen, covered with a layer of netting and heated to 105 degrees, then applied to the patient. The heat was maintained by applying a hot water bottle over the poultice (Oh, where were the Aqua-K pads back then?). The poultice was usually applied for 20 minutes every four hours. Lotions and liniments were also ordered and applied.

Pain medications when ordered were used very stringently. Pre-operative medications such as atropine and scopolamine and pain medications such as morphine were available only in tablet form.

Having checked the correct dose as ordered, the tablet was placed in a spoonful of water, heated over a Bunsen burner until dissolved, drawn up into a syringe and administered intra-muscularly. The only site used was the upper outer quadrant of the buttock. The site was ro-tated with each prescribed dose.

Patients with cerebral vascular accidents or pa-tients who were post-craniotomy, or in a comatose state were given nourishment by tube feeding. A rubber stomach tube, which was very thick, was inserted through the oral cavity three times a day.

Normal food like buttered bread, cooked meat, vegetables and fruit were ground up with a hand grinder, mixed with water and poured with a jug into a funnel attached to the stomach tube. Many of these patients remained in the hospital for months at a time. The stomach was checked for tube placement by injecting a little air into the tube and listening for sounds from the stomach with your ear.

A nurse from the day shift did urine testing each morning. The night nurse collected the necessary specimens early in the morning according to the physician's orders. Urine was tested for specific gravity, albumin, sugar and acetone. The results were documented in the patient's record. The specimens had to be accurately labeled and the nurse was always diligent not to mix up results.

Patients with diabetes had their urine tested before each meal and their insulin dose was titrated according to the results. Green was +1, yellow was +2, orange was +3 and brick red was

+4. If the urine was +3 or +4, it was also tested for acetone. (Ketone bodies). Thank God for modern day Accu-Cheks.

During my second year of training, I learned how to give enemas, do catheterizations and give insulin injections. The learning scale was hierarchical in nature. Third year nursing students were delegated more responsibility than second year students. Second year students had more responsibility than the first year students. Each student assisted those more junior to her with knowledge and shills. However, that did not always work, as I will share with you a little later.

In those days, pre-packaged medical kits were unavailable. Every thing was assembled, placed on a stainless steel tray, covered with a clean towel and taken to the patient's bedside. For instance, when giving an enema, I assembled the tray, a rubber rectal catheter, additional rubber tubing, and a jug of warm soapy water, a rubber sheet and a funnel.

On one occasion, the doctor's order was to give a "high soap suds enema." I asked a more senior student what "high" meant. She told me to stand on a stool. I have never figured out if she did not know or if she was putting me on.

Over the years, I have cared for many patients and have vivid memories. I remember one patient very well. He was a fifty-year-old man who was hit by a lorry (truck) while crossing a busy road. The Cork Dublin road was one of the busiest roads in Ireland at that time. I believe it still is. The man was a teacher and Hurling coach at a local school. He was in a comatose state when brought to the hospital. I was one of the nurses assigned to his care on the night shift. His bed was located in the corner of the male surgical ward. The curtains were drawn and black screens surrounded his bed to keep out light. Magnesium Sulfate enemas were ordered at two hourly intervals to relieve intracranial pressure. He hiccoughed constantly for ten days until he died. The night he died, I heard the Banshee cry.

The Banshee, in Irish folklore, was a female spirit whose cry was heard preceding the death of some families. One of my other patients told me that the dead man's mother was named McCarthy and that the Banshee cried after people who had O or Mc as a prefix to their name. When the man died, I heard a low, mournful wail that came from outside the ward. I was with another nurse and when she turned to me with a pale face and fright in her eyes, I knew that I did not imagine hearing the Banshee's cry.

The last part of our post-mortem care was removing the body from the ward and bringing it to a small chapel in the courtyard. We went through the steps with great hesitation. Neither of us wanted to make that trip out to the chapel and meet the Banshee. You can imagine the relief we felt when the Sister came to us and said that this time we could leave the body in the ward until morning. I then realized that she heard the Banshee too.

The post mortem examination (autopsy) revealed that the area of the brain that controlled hiccoughing, coughing, and sneezing, was destroyed by the accident. Hence, the reason for his uncontrolled hiccoughing.

On one occasion, a Norwegian merchant ship docked in Cork harbor. A crewmember was rushed to the hospital with acute appendicitis. After his surgery, the patient was cared for in the male surgical ward. We learned that the patient had a "picture" of a woman on his left buttock. The patient did not speak English, but on showing him the rectal thermometer, he obligingly turned over. When the nuns were in chapel, he had his temperature taken a great many times by curious staff. At that time, I naively believed the picture was a birthmark. I later learned about tattoos. Now, I know there is a need for HIPAA to protect patients!

I worked on a male urological floor where patients with bladder or prostate conditions had Foley urethral catheters or supra-pubic catheters. These catheters drained urine into a large glass jar at the bedside. We dubbed this ward "The Lily Pond". Dressing changes took all morning, and screens were moved and placed around the bed to insure privacy. The dressing cart had to be stocked and moved by the bed and the nurse had to drape the patient and then wash her hands in the sink at the end of the ward. During the dressing change, the procedure provided a good time to listen to the patient's concerns and reassure him as to his progress.

Intravenous therapy was unheard of but if a blood transfusion was required, the doctor started saline intravenously and the blood was then transfused over a six-hour period. Heaven help the nurse who "allowed" the IV to go subcutaneous, meaning the fluid leaked into the surrounding tissues. The doctor had to be called to restart it. Blood was provided in a glass bottle, which was warmed to 98.4 degrees before being transfused into the patient. We knew the blood types and the Rhesus factor but little else.

If a patient was dehydrated and was unable to take fluids by mouth, small quantities of a hypertonic saline solution was given subcutaneously into the abdominal wall over a four hour period. The site was changed every day and a drug named Varidase was injected into the site to increase absorption.

Back then, we never asked questions. We only did as the doctor ordered. As I mentioned before, nurses were considered "handmaidens of the doctors".

Each year consisted of one month in the classroom for what was called block training, seven months working rotating day shift in the different units, three months night duty and finally one-month vacation. During the night shift tour, I did not get any nights off. I worked from 7:00 p.m. to 8:30 a.m. with one hour off for supper. If quiet time was available during the night, I was expected to study. Also, many chores were assigned to the night shift, like mending hems and seams in the bed linen, and sanitizing bedpans, urinals and denture mugs. The urinals, bedpans and denture mugs were made of white enamel. When giving a bedpan or a urinal to a patient, it had to be covered and the bed was screened.

During the course of my nursing training, I observed death for the first time. It was a new experience for me and I began to cry. My instructor told me I would never make a nurse because I was too emotional. Fifty years later, I often cry when one of my patients passes on, sometimes in gratitude that their suffering is over, and often because I have grown fond of them.

Post mortem care was another skill I learned. Back in the 1950s, embalming was not available in Ireland. When a person died, the body was left untouched for one hour. The belief was to give the soul time to leave the body. The patient was then bathed, shaved if necessary and the body orifices were packed. The body was dressed in a brown garment called a habit, the eyes were closed and the hands crossed. I was taught that a dead person deserved as much respect as a living one. One occasion, I was involved in giving post mortem care to a person whose family's religious beliefs involved leaving the body untouched. I was unaware of this and again got in trouble and had to write a letter of apology to each family member.

I really enjoyed caring for children and had much rapport and patience with them. I was the youngest member of my family and did not have much involvement with younger children, so I considered it a novelty to care for them. One year I was very proud to receive a prize for being pediatric nurse of the year. However, in later years, when I was a mother I found it difficult to care for sick children.

The last year of training, I was assigned to the operating room. I learned the names of the instruments and the idiosyncrasies of the surgeons. I was a rotating nurse and then a scrub nurse assisting the surgeon. The nun in charge of the operating room was very strict and impatient. I must admit I was happy when my six-week rotation was completed. I disliked the tense atmosphere.

The hospital that I trained in no longer exists as such. The building was eventually sold and is now a Quality Inn hotel. A merchant in the city told me that it closed because there were no more nuns to run it. I figured the prayers of the student nurses over so many years were finally heard.

I recently visited there with some of my family and the beautiful Oak staircase is still there. My visit brought back some fond memories. When I told them I had been a student nurse there, I received the V.I.P. treatment and received a tour.

CHAPTER FOUR

When my general nursing training was completed and I was a state registered nurse, I decided to specialize in Midwifery. There was a long waiting list to get into maternity hospitals in Ireland, so I decided to travel to England for that particular training. The course consisted of one year of training. The first six months was spent in a maternity hospital. Once again, I was back in the classroom and the "Handbook of Maternity Nursing" became my bible. Classroom instruction was concurrent with the hands-on care.

The maternity clinic was affiliated with the hospital. Pregnant patients visited there for their monthly, biweekly, or weekly visits under the guidance of an obstetrician. Weight gain was monitored as was blood pressure and the testing of the urine for albumin on each clinic visit.

I learned how to palpate the abdomen, listen for fetal heart tones and do rectal and vaginal examinations. I had to relate my findings to the physician who did comparative examinations. The student midwife had to complete fifty examinations.

I remember on one occasion I examined a patient and proudly told the physician the baby was in a breech position. He sent me to retrieve a record of the patient's previous pregnancies. When I returned, he instructed me to re-examine the patient. This time I was very unsure of my finding because I found the baby was a cephalic presentation. The doctor was aware of my confusion and informed me he had manually rotated the fetus while I was away. The patient told me "he had pulled a fast one on me."

When a patient was admitted in labor, the midwives knew her from clinic visits and her prenatal records were available in anticipation of her arrival. The routine procedure was history of contractions, vital signs, physical examination, personal preparation and a soap suds enema if the membrane was still intact. The patient then received a warm tub bath. Labor was considered normal and deliveries were never rushed. Modern technology was unavailable back then, so I was taught to rely on observation skills and awareness of complications that could occur. Cesarean sections and episiotomies were rare occurrences.

I observed thirty deliveries, and then was allowed to assist the doctor or midwife with ten more. I was then ready to deliver my first baby under supervision however, this did not happen.

I happened to be on night duty when a primipara (first pregnancy) patient was admitted and the supervisor assigned me to her care. The patient told me her labor had started a few hours earlier and her contractions were mild and were 15 to 20 minutes apart. I proceeded with her care and assisted the patient into the bathtub. After a few minutes, the patient began to have painful contractions 1 to 2 minutes apart. Her face was red and she was pushing hard. I encouraged her to pant as I assisted her out of the tub. I can still feel that little head in the palm of my hand as I laid mom on the bath mat and delivered a beautiful baby girl. I yelled for help, which came immediately. The supervisor told me I did a wonderful job but I was in too much shock to believe her. That was the first of many deliveries for me.

I assisted at one delivery where the infant girl did not have digits in her left hand. The mother suffered the tragic loss of her father during early pregnancy, before she knew she was pregnant. The mother's girlfriend gave her a pill (sedative) to help her get over the trauma of the wake and funeral. It was determined that the medication taken was thalidomide. Around that time, many babies were delivered with birth defects traced to mothers being on the Thalidomide medication.

During my time as a midwife, I delivered breech and footling presentations, twins and one baby who had a papyraceus fetus attached to his shoulder.

I also learned how to care for the newborn baby. This involved bathing, dressing, feeding, burping and cord and eye care. I completed a tour of duty in the premature baby nursery. The infant was in a private room and two nurses covered the twenty-four hour period of care. This was done to decrease the number of people interacting with the baby. The parents were allowed to view their baby from the observation window and I always felt sad that they were unable to hold them.

The nurse double gowned, masked and gloved before entering the room. She then removed the outer layer in the room before caring for the infant. The temperature in the room was usually high. To prevent too much handling, the baby was left in the cot. The baby was cleaned, dressed and fed every one to two hours. Baby oil was applied to the skin daily and as needed.

Expressed breast milk was brought in from the mother and if the baby was too weak to suck, a pipette was used to drop the milk into the mouth. A quarter teaspoon of Nestlé's condensed milk was given four times a day to promote weight gain. The babies sucked very slowly from a special nipple but really enjoyed the taste of the condensed milk.

The nurses were encouraged to talk and sing to the babies, and gently massage them. We became very attached to these special babies and parted from them with mixed emotions. Happy that they had reached five pounds and were healthy enough to go home, but sad to see them leave. We lost an occasional few, which was always heartbreaking, but we had done our best for them.

During my tour of duty in Maternity Part One, I encountered one episode of post partum depression. I was caring for a patient who was five days post partum. When I brought the baby from the nursery for the evening nursing, the mother attempted to throw the baby on the floor. She yelled and screamed that she never had a baby and became very agitated and combative. The patient was discharged to a mental facility and the baby remained in the nursery until the family made appropriate arrangements for his care.

I was always in awe of the miracle of birth and felt privileged to be part of it. Having completed the Maternity Part One training and having passed the qualifying examination, I began Maternity Part Two. In those days 80% of births occurred in the home. The midwife, who cared for a patient in the prenatal clinic, was the midwife who attended the delivery. Some primipara patients, premature, and multiple births, were recommended for hospital delivery.

CHAPTER FIVE

Maternity Part Two nursing involved training the student midwife to participate in home births and care of the mother and infant after the birth.

Each student was assigned to a district midwife and worked with her in the prenatal and postnatal clinics and accompanied her to the home births in that district. The midwife was also responsible for the training and housing of the students assigned to her. Two students were usually assigned for a six-month time frame.

The midwife had her own car, but the students used a bicycle. When the call came in that the patient had started labor, the student rode her bike to the patient's home. The radius was usually about 5-6 miles. As you know a baby can be born anytime, but as a student midwife, I firmly believed that all babies arrived between 1:00 a.m. and 4:00 a.m.

About one month before the patients expected due date (EDD), the midwife dropped off a delivery pack. The pack consisted of a sterile sheet, towels, gloves, scissors, dressings and perineal pads. A rubber sheet was also included. We instructed the patient to save some newspapers for the occasion. The newspapers were placed under the sheet to protect the mattress

When I arrived at the home, I assessed the patient, reassured the dad and prepared the bed and patient for the delivery. We occasionally had false alarms but that is part of the story. Unlike what we see in the movies, everything was very relaxed and normal.

For me, one of the downsides was the low beds. I am tall and after the delivery, I usually ended up with a backache.

For the first ten deliveries, the midwife was present and observed the delivery and my care of the mother and baby. After that, I was on my own. I guess I was never on my own because I constantly invoked the help of God, the Blessed Virgin and a host of angels and saints to help me.

After the delivery, I returned to the patient's home two times daily for the first three days and once a day for seven more days. I monitored the vital signs, level of the fundus and the color and amount of the uterine discharge. The mother was encouraged to rest in the Fowler's position for a few hours each day as this helped with uterine discharge.

I instructed the mother how to bathe and dress the baby, how to breast feed, prepare formula and how to sterilize bottles and nipples. The mother and baby were discharged on the tenth day under normal circumstances. The mother brought the baby to the clinic at three weeks and six weeks for weighting and general observation. At the six-week check up, the mother was discharged until the next pregnancy.

The system of home birth was carefully monitored. The closest district hospital had a "Flying Squad" available to bring immediate care to the home should an emergency occur. The flying squad consisted of an obstetrician, another doctor, a laboratory technician and a midwife. The midwife at the home called the hospital for help if needed.

The ambulance with the team arrived at the home within ten or fifteen minutes. The mother or baby was given the necessary first aide and was transported to the hospital as quickly as possible. It was a relief to know that assistance was readily available. Each hospital's flying squad had seven minutes to be in the ambulance from the time the emergency call came in. The necessary equipment was always packed and the ambulance was always on standby.

One night, I was on my way to a patient's house when I encountered a drunken man. It was about 2:00 a.m. and I was pushing my bike up a hill. The man recognized me as a nurse and offered to push my bike for me. I was worried that he would steal the bike and I would not make the birth in time. I told him I was in a rush, hopped on my bike and began to pedal furiously. He wished me good luck and said he wanted to help. I appreciated his good intentions. We were much safer back then. We were recognized as nurses by our uniforms and respected for our nursing qualifications.

After completing the second portion of my midwifery training and passing the qualifying examination I was officially declared a State Certified Midwife (SCM).

I decided to continue working as a midwife and found employment in a maternity clinic in London. Many of the patients were poor migratory workers who literally walked in off the street to have their babies delivered. Most of them had no prenatal care. I was one of six midwives who worked the day shift 7:00 a.m. to 7:00 p.m. The first midwife on duty took the first patient and we rotated throughout the day and helped each other out as necessary.

There was really teamwork involved because on busy days we really needed each other to survive. One day, I delivered nine babies including twins. I remember on one occasion, a neighboring hospital emergency room called that they were sending over a patient who had come in with abdominal pain.

She said she had eaten cabbage the day before and it usually gave her gas pains. I delivered her baby on the ambulance cart. She didn't know she was pregnant. There was never a dull moment.

On another occasion, a patient told me she gave birth to her previous baby while working in a field and that she just squatted down and delivered. Our procedure at that time was to have the patient lay in the left lateral position. This position gave the midwife more control of the delivery and prevented trauma to the perineum. I have since learned that this is referred to as the English Method. My patient wanted no part in my positioning strategy and I had no alternative but to concur with her wishes. The result was an easy delivery of a healthy baby with no trauma to the mother. I learned that day that rules are made to be broken.

I remember another woman who presented to the clinic in strong labor, with contractions occurring at regular intervals. She gave a history of Gravida XV11 (seventeenth pregnancy) and a Para X11 (twelve live birth deliveries). In my ignorance, I believed she would deliver instantly as I hustled her into the delivery room. Over the course of the day, her contractions wore off and the fetal heart tones dropped. The patient ended up having an emergency caesarean section. She had uterine inertia; her uterus was too worn out for normal labor to progress.

After delivery, patients were transferred to the adjoining hospital for the usual post partum care. I worked there for a year and gained such valuable experience. My next position as a midwife was in a Jewish Maternity hospital. It was a very happy atmosphere. After the baby boys were born, the Rabbi circumcised them on the eighth day.

There was a special room available for this ceremonial event. One time, I took the baby to the room and attempted to stay but the Rabbi told me to leave. As a gentile I did not belong. The midwife who had delivered the baby was usually assigned to cleaning the room after the ceremony. She always found pastries and wine there. These items were readily confiscated to the midwives' quarters for a party that night. We usually dubbed it "circumcision wine". I came to believe that those goodies were left there intentionally for us. We were very happy when the baby boys were born.

CHAPTER SIX

When I first went to England in the late 1950s, I met many people from other countries; most of them were British subjects. I enjoyed learning about their backgrounds and cultures. However, I had difficulty accepting their different religious beliefs. When I grew up in the South of Ireland, my country was then over ninety percent Roman Catholic and I had never been exposed to anything else. I remember working with peers and thinking "She is so nice and she is a Protestant". I could not equate the two.

Over the years, I have developed friendships with wonderful people of many religious denominations and have benefited from the experience. I had a friend who lived in the North of England and she invited me home for a weekend to hear the Reverend Billy Graham speak. He was visiting there from the United States. Hearing the word of God so eloquently expressed left an awesome impression on me. I shared my experience with my mother who told me "I was losing my religion". Over the years, I have continued to embrace the faith of my ancestors but I realize that others are also entitled to their own-beliefs.

A few years ago, I was invited to a Bar Mitzvah and my friend Jake said it was a miracle to see an Irish Catholic in a synagogue on Christmas Eve. Later, during a sad period in my life, I received advice and consolation from a Rabbi friend that still provides me with comfort.

After some time, I decided to return to general nursing. I worked in the London Clinic as a private duty nurse. I was assigned to one patient and usually worked a twelve-hour shift. Back then, many people travelled from Greece, Turkey and South Africa for orthopedic procedures. Family usually accompanied the patient. They usually stayed in a suite of rooms adjacent to the patient. Family members, though concerned, were very agreeable not to interfere with the nurse's routine when caring for the patient. They visited at meal-times to provide socialization or if the patient requested company.

The daily routine consisted of waking the patient at seven in the morning, providing early morning care, breakfast, bathing, and doing dressing changes and exercises recommended by the surgeon. The patient could read or take a short nap if he so desired. At 11:00 a.m., the patient received light nourishment and had family visit for a short interval. A housekeeper was assigned to room cleaning and the kitchen staff served all meals.

When the patient was napping, the nurse could read, knit or relax and listen to the radio. (No TV back then). After lunch, the patient had more exercises and could visit with family and friends. 3:00 p.m. brought afternoon tea and the patient was encouraged to take another nap. It was believed that healing occurred during sleep. While the patient had his early afternoon nap, I could go out for two hours to walk shop or meet friends. The family was aware of this and another nurse was always on call for emergencies, should they arise. At 5:00 p.m., the patient had a dressing change if needed, evening care consisting of skin care and oral hygiene. Supper was usually served at 6 p.m. After supper, the patient could have visitors until 8 p.m. He was then prepared for bedtime.

During that period, I met many wonderful people. One Turkish family gave me coffee in a beautiful demitasse cup at eleven each morning. I can still recall how delicious it was and how it gave me energy for the rest of the day. I took care of a titled gentleman from South Africa whose wife visited him each afternoon and his mistress came in the evening. At least, that is who he said they were. I do know they were not casual acquaintances.

The London Clinic was well known for its excellent care and for the titled and famous people who visited there. One of my coworkers told me she had cared for Elizabeth Taylor when she had a tracheotomy there.

CHAPTER SEVEN

After many months, I decided to move on but for a long time I missed the sound of Big Ben. A nurse friend and I decided to spend a summer at a seaside resort in the south of England. Nursing positions were readily available at many private nursing homes there.

Private nursing homes were for the wealthy patients who did not want to be cared for in general hospitals under socialized medicine. I got a position as a night supervisor and my friend Beth worked the day shift. We worked four days/nights on and three off. We occasionally had the same time off. On one such occasion, we bought tanning lotion (new on the market) and applied it to each other. On returning to work, we told our co-workers we had gone to the European continent to sunbathe. About two hours into my shift, I had to scrub for an emergency herniorrhaphy. Between that and the generous mopping of my forehead by the circulating nurse, my tan quickly disappeared.

When winter came, I decided to return to London and return to general nursing in a large hospital. I was employed as a charge nurse in a surgical ward. I was addressed as "sister," the title given to a nurse in charge. It had no religious connotation. It took me a long time to get accustomed to it. Staff nurses and students were assigned to my ward. It was a very busy place as we had surgical patients arriving all the time.

Surgeon's rounds occurred each morning. Surgical residents, interns and medical students accompanied the surgeon. The ward sister (me) and a staff nurse accompanied them with the patients' record and a dressing cart. Sister gave a brief history of the patient, including name age, diagnosis, vital signs and appearance of the wound. These rounds took a long time, depending on the number of patients assigned to that particular surgeon. If the surgeon gave specific orders, sister documented them in her notebook and later transferred them to the patient's record as verbal orders. We were now using sulfa drugs and penicillin was available but not often prescribed.

I really enjoyed working there and believed I had found my niche, until one morning when I was summoned to Matron's office. I wondered what I had done wrong! She informed me I was assigned to work in the venereal disease clinic for the next three months. The person in charge had an emergency appendectomy during the night and I was to replace her. I was in shock. I mumbled that I knew nothing about VD. She assured me I would do fine since I had good managerial skills. One did not argue with Matron.

Early the next morning, I was given the keys to the clinic. The doctors and nursing staff quickly filled me in on what was expected of me. At that time, prostitution was legal in England. However, the prostitute was expected to take care of herself and was required to report to VD clinics for routine examinations, treatments and medication if necessary. Syphilis and Gonorrhea were the only known venereal diseases at that time. The "girls" received douches and medications as prescribed by the clinic physician.

On one occasion, one of the girls told me I worked too hard and that she would make more money that night than I would make in six months. I agreed with her but told her that I was needed to care for her on her return visits. To each to his own! I was happy to turn over the keys to the regular charge nurse but I missed the weekends off.

CHAPTER EIGHT

I transferred to a medical ward and found the pace much slower. The patients were hospitalized for longer periods of time. In those days, we received numerous patients with respiratory illnesses. Many had spent years working in the coalmines and the London smog was horrific. This resulted in many recurrent bouts of respiratory failure.

The oxygen was contained in large tanks that we hauled to the patients' bedside. The tank was elevated in a heavy metal stand and chained to the wall to prevent it from falling. Piped in oxygen was unavailable and there were no respiratory therapists. We gave respiratory treatments including postural drainage. For postural drainage, the patient was placed in the head and chest down position and kept that way for fifteen to twenty minutes.

Percussion was performed by cupping ones hands over a patient's ribcage and gently tapping. This technique assisted in lung drainage in patients with lung abscess and bronchiectasis. We did this procedure at least every six hours.

Oxygen tents were available for infants and children with respiratory conditions. I also cared for patients with poliomyelitis. The patients who had paralysis of the chest muscles and had difficulty breathing were placed in an Iron Lung (Tank respirator). This tank could maintain breathing artificially until the patient could do so independently. The sides of the tank had portal windows, which allowed the nurse to reach in and adjust the patient's limbs or bedclothes.

All large hospitals had an emergency flying squad (EFS), to which I was assigned at one time. The EFS responded to causalities that occurred in the community. Emergency supplies were always ready with an ambulance on stand-by. The doctors and nurses assigned to the team were in the ambulance within seven minutes of the call.

On time, the EFS were called to a train wreck. The smog was so dense the ambulance followed two men holding a white sheet and lanterns to the accident scene. Fortunately, another hospital that was closer to the scene got there faster. The train collision had occurred due to the smog. On subsequent visits to London, I was happy to see the smog isn't as bad due to better pollution control.

At that time, the hospital offered to send me to the University of London on a scholarship for medical training. I had gone through many years of studying and was not ready to commit to more. I was grateful but refused the offer.

CHAPTER NINE

I decided to return home to Ireland to work. A new sanitarium had opened up in a city near my home and I went to work there. Back then, Ireland was a very poor country with large families and poor housing conditions. The damp cold climate was also a factor as was poor nutrition. Tuberculosis (TB) was very prevalent. In this sanitarium, whole families were institutionalized with active TB. This was usually pulmonary but the germ invaded other organs also. A close friend of mine had an emergency laparotomy. Her great omentum was infected with the tuberculin bacilli.

It was truly amazing how cheerful these patients were. They had deep religious convictions.

They accepted their illness as God's will. To pass the time, they attended movies, did arts and crafts, read and prayed. I still have a beautiful leather bible cover made by one of my patients.

I was fortunate enough to work there when Ionized, Para Amino Salicylic Acid (PAAS) and streptomycin were discovered to be drugs of choice in the treatment of TB. Within months, we saw the miracle of healing. Sputum specimens became negative for growth and pulmonary lesions healed. However not all patients responded to the drugs. After three months of negative sputum specimens and chest x–rays, patients were discharged home on medication for at least one year. All sanitariums were closed in the early nineteen seventies and the disease is rarely if ever diagnosed anymore in that country.

A separate wing of that hospital was used for cardiac experimentation. Greyhounds were considered to have hearts similar to humans, so cardiac surgeons worked on them in an attempt to correct structural defects. The hounds were well cared for and received adequate medication. I was strongly opposed to these surgeries, partly because when I was younger, my brother raised greyhounds and I really loved those puppies. Today when I see the tremendous results from these interventions and the benefit to humanity, I think differently.

CHAPTER TEN

In 1961, my sister Margaret invited me to visit her in Chicago. An Uncle advised me to get an Emigrant Visa instead of a visitor's visa. He said the former would give me more freedom to work if I wished to explore nursing here. I visited with family and friends for about a month.

While in Chicago, I read an advertisement for a nurse at a local hospital. I applied at the hospital and obtained a staff position in the Labor and Delivery unit. I felt this was my forte and that delivering babies was the same the world over. The Director of Nurses hired me as a foreign graduate nurse. I earned three hundred dollars per month. She informed me that if I was registered in the State of Illinois, my salary would increase by fifty dollars but advised me to work in my present capacity for one year. I worked the day shift, which consisted of ten-hour days and six days per week. After a few months, I received my RN by reciprocity, as my previous training was more than adequate. I worked at that hospital for almost one year but never did receive the raise. I was never comfortable in the environment. Everyone was in a hurry all the time.

Nurses who had worked there many years claimed ownership to the hospital and spoke a language other than English in my presence. In the United Kingdom, I was unaware of prejudice. I had interacted with people of various ethnic backgrounds. I had worked with many Europeans and people from the British Colonies, the West Indies, Jamaica and Hong Kong. I had never experienced hostility before. I planned to return to Ireland but my family advised me to work in another hospital before going back.

I moved on to a newer and larger hospital in the southwest suburbs of Chicago. When I first worked there, I thought it was large in comparison to European hospitals. The hospital has since grown to about five times its original size. I felt welcome and appreciated there.

I worked in medical, surgical, orthopedic and pediatric units and for the first time I worked with married nurses who had returned to work after motherhood. I returned to Ireland to visit my family but I yearned for the large modern hospital where I had so much to learn. I worked as a head nurse and supervisor.

I attended the University of St. Francis in Joliet, Illinois for further degrees. The opportunities for continuing education were so vast in this country in comparison to Europe at that time and many nurses were taking advantage of them.

I also became certified in Cardio Pulmonary Resuscitation (CPR) and in First Aid. I later taught some home care classes for the American Red Cross and taught CPR to numerous Boy Scout and Girl Scout troops. I am very proud that both my sons are Eagle Scouts and my daughter is a Gold Award recipient. I believe that everyone possible should have CPR training. I have personally performed CPR in a fabric store, on a bus and in church. It never hurts to be prepared.

Back in the 1960s, nursing students earned a nursing diploma after three years of studying but times were changing. Hospitals being affiliated with universities and four-year degree nursing programs were becoming popular. Some community colleges were offering 2 year nursing programs and hospitals also employed licensed practical nurses (LPN) and nurse aides (NA).

The hospital opened its first Intensive Care Unit. I was appointed head nurse of the four-bed unit. One registered nurse and one nurse aide were assigned to the unit each shift. Hemodynamic monitoring was not yet available there. My first four patients were burn victims who were working in a nearby factory that caught fire. Two patients were critical and two were considered serious. They were three brothers and a cousin. Dressings were changed frequently and they received intravenous therapy for fluid replacement. I had to assign another nurse to help with their care, as the dressings were very time consuming.

All four patients had frequent debridement and skin graft surgeries. As time passed, their conditions improved and they were transferred to the regular floor. Postoperative care now consisted of intravenous therapy and nurses were taught how to insert IV needles and intercatheters. However, we timed the drops with our watch and we knew exactly how many drops per minute for a four-hour bottle.

No IVAC's or calculators back then. Sometimes they ran too fast or too slow and they had to be monitored frequently. All too often, we heard "The bottle is empty". As technology advanced, nursing care had to keep up and new techniques were constantly developed.

The hospital consisted of two, three and four bed units and patient care was conducted with greater privacy. Curtains suspended from the ceiling could be pulled around each bed. I never missed the old screens that I pulled around the ward. The units were quieter and patients of the same age and diagnoses were put together.

Nurses now worked eight-hour shifts and forty-hour weeks and the concept of team nursing came into play. My surgical ward had thirty-six beds and was always full. Sometimes patients were held in the emergency room while waiting for a patient to be discharged and the bed cleaned and made up. The ward had two teams; each consisted of one RN, one LPN and two NAs. A medicine nurse also worked between both teams.

You must realize that in the sixties and seventies many fewer medicines were prescribed or available. The head nurse did rounds with the doctors and carried out the orders. All orders were hand written and carbon paper was routinely used to make copies. When the addressograph arrived, I witnessed another miracle.

I remember on one occasion a consulting surgeon requested a carbon paper insert for his notes. The paper was inadvertently turned upside-down (not by me this time). When he removed the bottom copy and realized what had happened, he was very upset. He said nothing but if looks could kill, I wouldn't be writing this book. Now we have copy machines and I have not seen a scrap of carbon paper in decades. Thank God.

The team RN did rounds, dressings and treatments, while the LPN assisted with baths transfers and helped the RN as needed. The NAs did vital signs, made beds and transported patients off the unit for tests and x-rays. When a patient went to surgery, a nurse and an aide accompanied her and upon discharge, the nurse aide took the patient downstairs. As you can visualize a lot of running around off the floor took place. Now hospitals employ transportation technicians who safely transport patients by cart or wheelchair to and from scheduled procedures.

The medication nurse gave all the pre-op medications and pain medications and was responsible for picking up the narcotics from the pharmacy and locking them in a double locked cabinet. She also counted the narcotics with the oncoming shift medication nurse. The number of each narcotic was entered in the narcotic book and cosigned by each nurse. When picking up the narcotics from the pharmacy, the nurse took the book with her and the pharmacist signed it. The keys to the narcotic cabinet were kept in the RN's possession at all times.

A nurse's worst nightmare was taking the narcotic keys home. They had to be returned to the hospital immediately and one or both locks had to be changed for security reasons. I believe many nurses were guilty of that error. Of course, we were all the way home when the phone call came. No cell phones back then!

Now we have the wonderful PYXIS. This automatic medication-dispensing device interfaces with the pharmacy computer system. The physician's orders are reviewed by the RN, faxed to the pharmacist and verified. The medications are readily available to the nurse and there is quick access for stat orders. This system also provides more security and accountability for controlled substances.

I thought I had remembered all aspects of the good old days of the Med Pass, but I forgot the Med Cards. These were small oblong cards about the size of a credit card. The patient's name, room and bed number and the name and dose of each medication was hand written on each card. The cards were color coded for the different times for administration. Green was daily, pink was BID, yellow was TID, blue was QID and grey was PRN.

There was a special rack on the medicine room wall where the cards were stacked under the various room and bed numbers (624-1). The physicians' medication orders were hand written into the medication kardex and were yellowed out when discontinued. The med cards were then made out from the kardex. The med nurse checked the med cards against the kardex at the beginning of each shift. We also had a treatment kardex and the treatment cards were white. If a

card was misplaced or was illegible, the physician'
order was reviewed and a new card was made.

Reflecting on the process, I can only say it was
tedious and time consuming. Shift notes had to
be made in different color ink for different shifts,
black for days, green for PM's and red for nights.

Now in modern times, we log into the computer, bring up each patient's name and read the
electronic medication administration record (E-
MAR). All the medications listed for the day, including the time due and when last given are
reviewed at a glance. What a time saver!

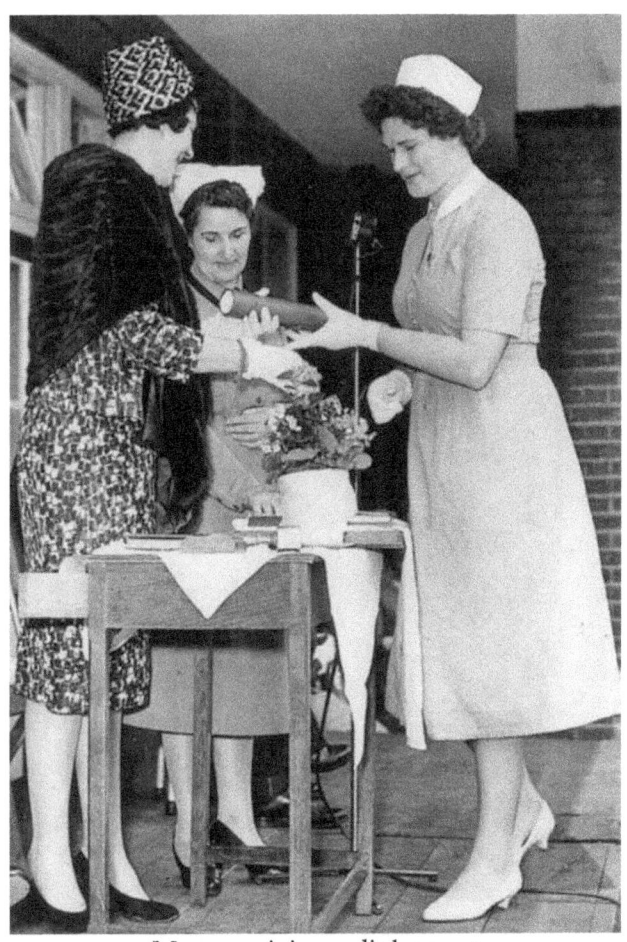

Mary receiving a diploma at
"Maternity Part I Graduation"

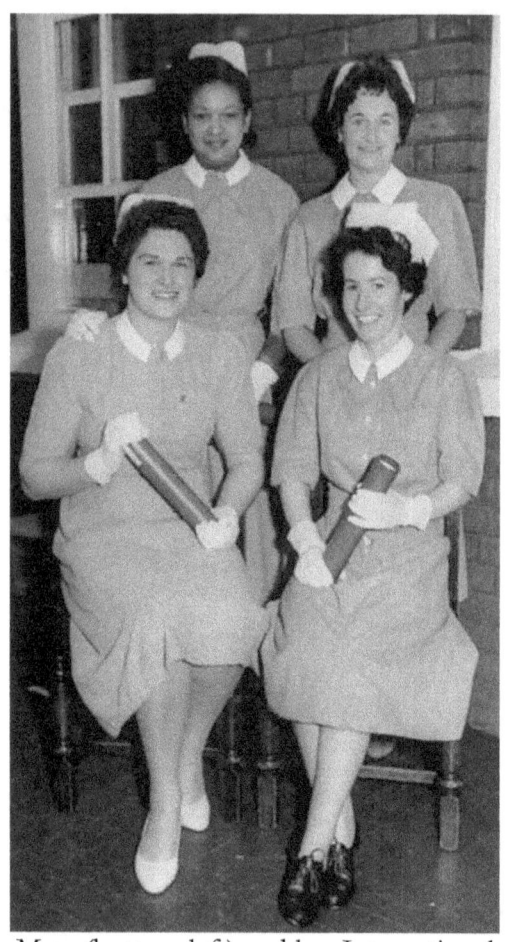

Mary (bottom left) and her International
friends representing Ireland, England,
Wales and the West Indies

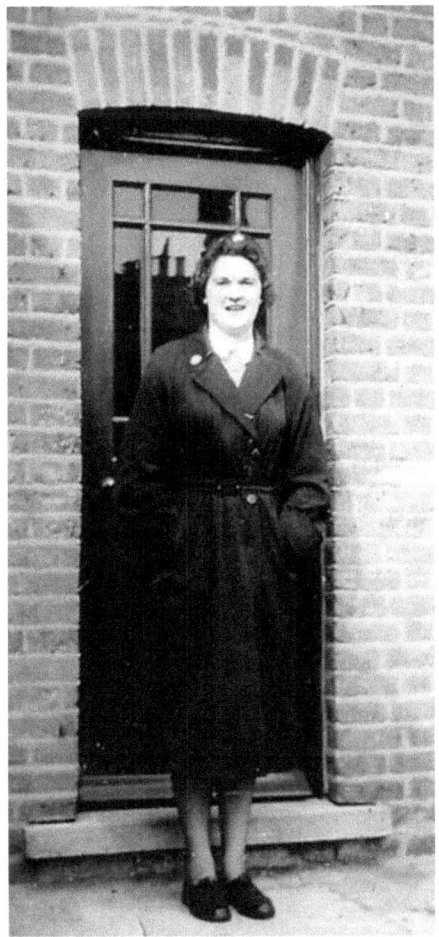

Mary in her outdoor nurse uniform

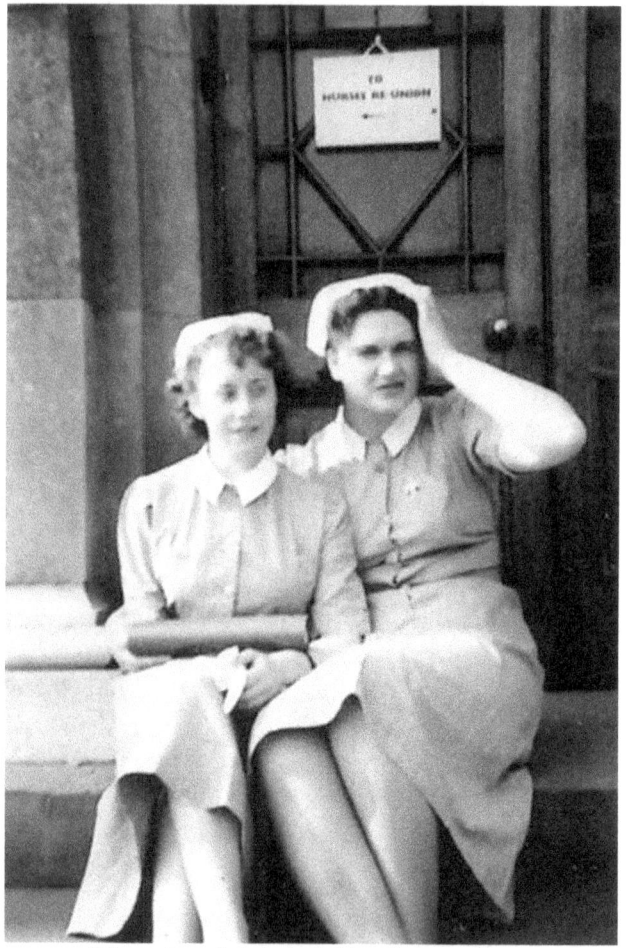

Mary (on right) and friend attending a
Nurse Reunion

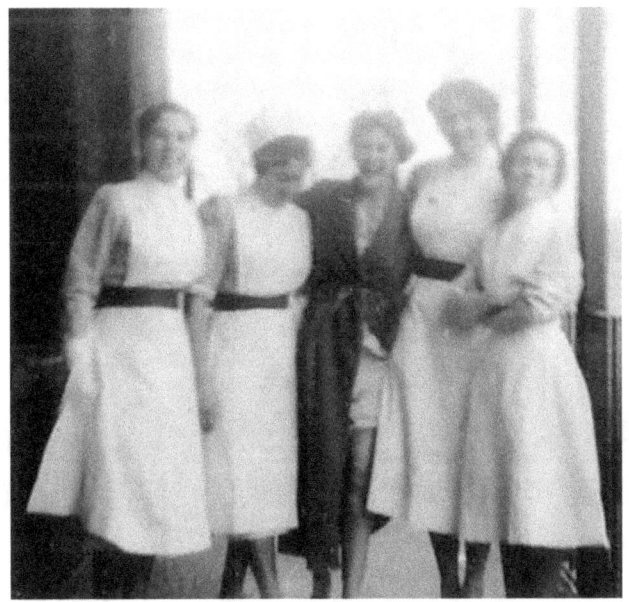

Mary (second from right) with friends at a
Nurse Reunion

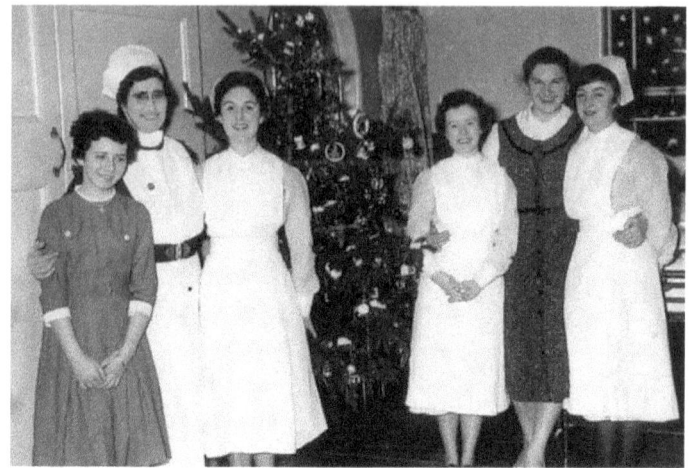

Mary (second from right) attending a Christmas Party
on her ward, during her day off.

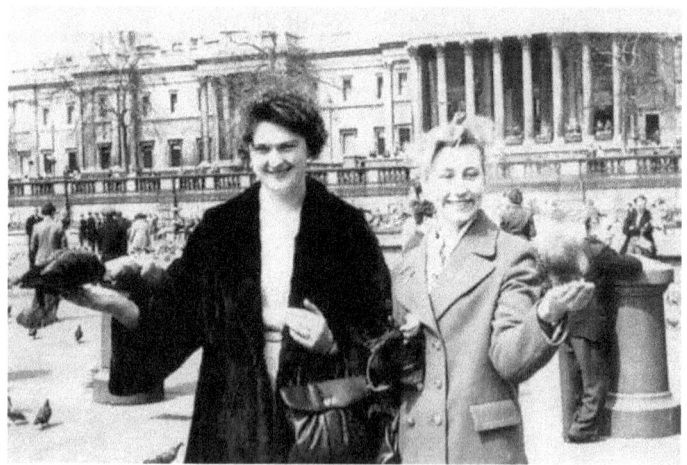

Mary and friend at Trafalgar Square in London

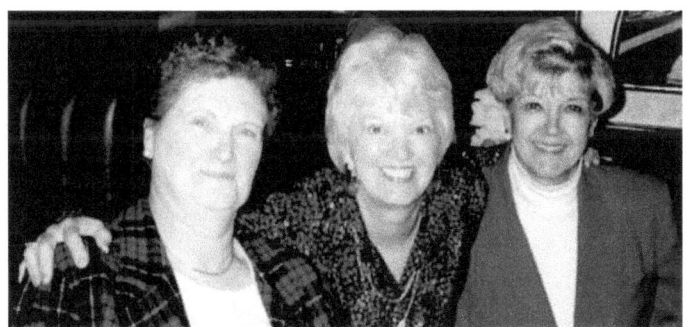

Mary with colleagues from HCFA

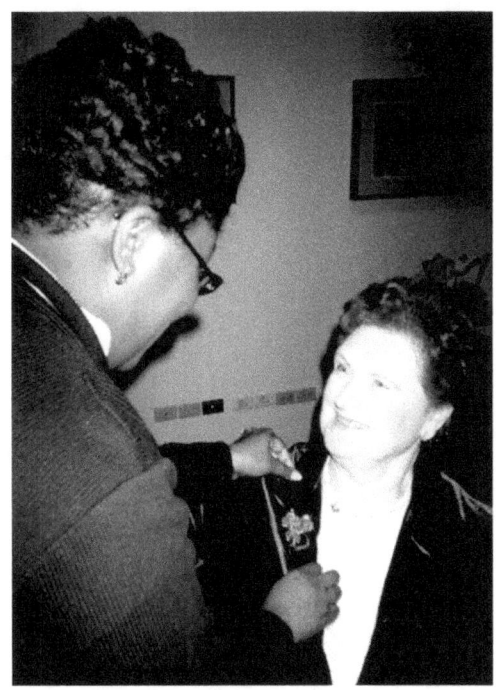

Mary receiving a pin at her
HCFA retirement party

CHAPTER ELEVEN

In the late 1960s, the hospital employed ward secretaries to assist with the transcribing of orders and running errands to other departments. This was very beneficial to the Head Nurse as she now only reviewed the orders and signed the order sheets. I must say that doctors' handwriting in general has not improved greatly over the years. However, there are some with great penmanship.

I remember on one occasion reviewing a patient's chart where the doctor had written the admitting diagnosis as "GOK". I had to track down the doctor to decipher that diagnosis. He told me "God only knows". I do not believe that would pass any insurance company in these times of preapproval. Another order I remember was "if no BM in PM give EM in AM". I figured that one out by myself.

Doctors were not readily available as they are today. Back then, there were no cell phones or pagers and we often had to wait a long time to receive a response. Office nurses guarded the doctor as fastidiously as did the doctors' wives. Sometimes it was very frustrating waiting for a call back.

Central supply was available for sterilizing of dressings and equipment. Syringes and needles were now disposable. Plastic became available and we became more aware of infection control. I attended an in-service on colostomy care using a disposable kit and colostomy bags and I thought I was in heaven.

Kits were available for dressing trays, catheterization trays and various irrigation trays. Nasogastric tubes and PEG (percutaneous endoscopic gastrostomy) tubes could remain in place for longer periods. Formulas became available as nutritional support. The nurses' life was becoming easier or so we believed.

During that time, I met my husband and had three children. I still worked part time on the weekends when my husband was home. I frequently visited Ireland and was happy to learn that health care had improved there also. The nurses now worked a forty-hour week and appropriate equipment was more readily available.

Based on my background as I have described in previous chapters, I was astonished at the progress in nursing and felt grateful to be part of such wonderful advances in the healthcare field. Throughout all aspects of my nursing career, I felt lucky to be a nurse and help relieve or alleviate the suffering of others. I learned about patience and fortitude from those whom I cared for.

Over the years, I've had many wonderful co-workers, who have given themselves constantly in the care and service of others. Nurses receive little thanks but we are not in the profession for accolades. Often, outcomes are not as we would like them to be but when things get tough, we are always there to support of one another and that makes it all worthwhile. It would be remiss of me if I did not mention the many wonderful nurses who were very close friends who are no longer with us. Many times, they had more courage than I had. I believed they were a great loss to the nursing profession and to patients they could have continued to care for and that they had gone before their time. However, that is not for me to say but I am sure they continue to provide great joy in their present surroundings.

One of my greatest experiences has been with patients as they transitioned from this life to the next. It has been so profound and I hope I have been of some help at that time by my presence, touch or prayer.

In the spring of 1967, a tornado touched down in our community causing unbelievable loss of life, severe bodily injuries and tremendous structural damage. I had not experienced that type of weather in the past and I remember feeling very scared. At that time, I was a head nurse in the orthopedic wing of the hospital and on the emergency call list.

My husband accompanied me to the hospital. We had to walk some of the way as there were trees and electrical wires down and it was unsafe to drive. I was assigned to triage and was kept very busy for several hours.

I assisted with contacting other hospitals in the area in an attempt to locate missing persons. It was heartbreaking to advise families to check in at the local VFW hall, which had been set up as a temporary morgue.

The next day when I returned to work, I found my orthopedic unit over flowing with patients who had been victims of the tornado. Over the next several months, nurses cared for many patients with not only serious physical injuries but also mental anguish caused by loss of family and friends and loss or damage to personal property.

Many of our patients suffered from crush injuries and gas gangrene. The patients received Hyperbaric Oxygen treatments (HBOT). The high volume of oxygen was used with the necessary orthopedic surgery and antibiotics. The HBOT helped decrease complications and as the increased oxygen was delivered to the injured tissue, swelling decreased and wound healing was aided with less infection as a result.

In the cases of gas gangrene, the high volume of oxygen hampered the bacterial growth and their ability to spread and make more toxins. Repeated HBOT helped to slow the progress of the infection, allowing surgery to remove the affected tissue and antibiotics to control the infection.

The use of traction has decreased over the years, but back then, patients with fractures were treated with traction. Cervical traction, Russell traction and Buck's traction were used to treat many patients with injuries and fractures acquired during the tornado. Our beds were fitted with overhead traction frames. After the traction was applied, the nursing challenge began. Correct alignment was of the utmost importance. The appropriate amount of weight and the changing of the patient's position were based on the physician's directive. Traction was applied for weeks or months and nursing care took much longer. Bathing and bed changing took two nurses as proper alignment and the free fall of the weights had to be maintained at all times.

Site care of the pins, wires, or tongs was done frequently and neurovascular checks were performed by a nurse at least every shift. Skin care was a serious challenge due to immobility and the risk of pressure sores occurring was high. We certainly not did have any of the wonderful beds or treatments available at present, not only to treat but also to prevent pressure sores. Another problem back then was that pain management was not readily available and as nurses, we had to rely on various alternatives to keep the patient comfortable.

During this time, we relied heavily on two pieces of equipment I have not seen in recent use. These were a Stryker frame and a Circle-electric bed. The frame sandwiched the patient between two strong pieces of material. One was anterior and one posterior to the patient's body.

The device was rotated along the long axis of the patient, which permitted positioning without motion of individual parts. The position was changed every two hours and when the patient was in the prone position a flap of material was released to allow the face to be free. The patient always felt scared and restless in this position. The positioning and general nursing care was time consuming and the patient was always changed to the recumbent position at mealtimes to be fed.

The circle-electric bed was also used to relieve pressure and to change the patient's position without hurting him or her. This bed was electric and enclosed between two circles. The patient was strapped in and when a button was pressed the bed rotated completely from the supine to the prone position. Again, the patient felt uncomfortable in a suspended state.

I can clearly visualize these two pieces of equipment but God failed to provide me with a talent for drawing. I cannot draw a straight line without a ruler. I feel so grateful for the wonderful beds that are now available for the patients' comfort and repositioning.

In the mid to late 1960s, Medicare and Medicaid spawned a tremendous growth in hospital and nursing home facilities. I remember one patient in particular who was in traction for a fractured femur and remained in the hospital for nine months. Many patients also developed an attitude that their continued hospitalization paid the nurses' salaries and we should be grateful. I believe that attitude dissipated with time.

CHAPTER TWELVE

In the early 1970s, the hospital where I worked decided to have an Intravenous Therapy Team as the physicians ordered IV fluids more frequently. At that time, we were known as the Venoclyses team. I received training on venous access and the maintenance of intravenous fluids.

A new era for nurses was evolving and we were considered very special to be able to do what only physicians did previously.

I worked the night shift. The IV therapy nurse did the initial start orders and was responsible for all transfusion orders. I picked up the units of blood from the blood bank where I checked it with the laboratory technician, rechecked it with the floor RN and proceeded to hang it. The floor RN was responsible for monitoring vital signs and observing for transfusion reactions.

I vividly remember one night (July 3, 1974) we had a patient in ICU who required many transfusions. At least five times, I paged the lab technician to meet me in the blood bank. It was one of those nights when the ER was full and everyone was extremely busy. My last page for him was about 6:00am. At that time, he was busy doing blood draws and he threatened to lock me up in the blood bank and I would be listed among the missing.

Occasionally, I was called to the Emergency Room to restart infiltrated (subcutaneous) IV's. We mainly used butterfly needles, which could dislodge easily. The least enjoyable part of my job was starting IV fluids in the pediatric department or using scalp veins in babies. The physicians usually ordered daily IV's, as heplocks were unavailable in those days.

Many of my coworkers called me "Mary Veno" and on one occasion, I met a former patient in a store who greeted me as "Mrs. Veno."

A few years later, the hospital discontinued the IV Therapy team as it was not cost effective and more staff nurses became proficient at starting IV's.

IV's where a needle is inserted and then taped to the skin are no longer used. The needles were replaced by catheters, which are thin flexible tubes that stay in the vein. Presently the catheters are available in different sizes and have shielding, making them easier to insert and maintain. Based on facility policy, a catheter can remain in place at least three or four days.

When a patient requires intravenous fluids or antibiotics over an extended period of time, a surgeon can insert a central line catheter. A peripherally inserted central catheter (PICC) can be inserted by a team of specially trained RN's. These lines can be used to give treatments such as antibiotics, intravenous fluids, chemotherapy and hyper alimentation. They can also be used to take samples of blood for testing. This is very beneficial as it saves on venipuncture, especially if veins are hardened or difficult to find.

Modern technology has produced a device to find veins called a venoscope. This allows the nurse to locate hard to find veins more quickly and easily. Fewer sticks are involved and the nurse has to spend less time with the patient and fewer supplies such as catheters, syringes and kits are wasted. The procedure is safer and more comfortable for the patient. In most circumstances, veins are easily located, but there are those patients with hard to find veins such as the obese, elderly, or dark-skinned patients. I wish the venoscope were available when I was Mary Veno.

In the early 1980s, I had the opportunity to work 12-hour shifts in the Intensive Care Unit for one year while completing a University program. I believed this was an excellent way to be home during the week with my family and attend classes. I worked from 7:00am to 7:00pm every Saturday and Sunday. Unfortunately, Christmas Eve and Christmas Day, New Year's Eve and New Years Day fell on Saturday and Sunday that year.

I felt sad being away from my family on those occasions and of course, I worked on Mother's Day and Easter Sunday. Based on that, I realized it wasn't such a wonderful idea after all; however I was committed to complete the year.

I was amazed at how Intensive Care Nursing had developed over the years. Advanced medical and surgical technology demanded corresponding increase in bedside nursing techniques and as I have previously mentioned, nurses are always learning. The original nurses training is but the first step in a lifetime of acquiring new knowledge and skills. The Intensive Care Unit I worked in had progressed to hemodynamic monitoring, pacemaker insertion and Swanz-Ganz catheters. We had now learned Cardio Pulmonary Resuscitation (CPR) and codes for response to emergencies in the hospital were initiated.

From a nursing standpoint, it was difficult to continue patient care on the weekends. I firmly believe in continuity of care when possible. It is better for both the patient and nurse. Too much had occurred over the course of a week. It was difficult to keep up with the results of tests and x-rays performed during the week. All reports were hard copy. We did not have computerized records back then. Now all pertinent information is available at the click of a mouse.

In General Nursing care, the ratio of nurse to patients is usually 1:8, but in the ICU the ratio is much lower because of the patient's acuity. Our staffing load consisted of one patient if critically ill, or two to three if less acute. One would believe that caring for a few patients was not a heavy assignment, but it is amazing how much care is involved and how important observations and good nursing judgment are, as a patient's condition can change instantaneously.

I was happy when my one-year assignment was complete and I returned to less strenuous and demanding work. As I described in an earlier chapter on my training experience in the operating room, I believe my personality is geared to a more predictable type of care. However, I am always willing to push myself and gain additional experience.

After completing my work in Intensive Care, I decided to specialize in Long Term Care nursing which quickly became a new love in my life. Caring for the elderly is truly an awesome experience. Over the course of their long lives they have experienced so much pain, suffering and hardships, they are truly entitled to all the care and nurturing we can provide for them. I became a night supervisor in a large skilled care nursing home. Back then, there was a huge stigma attached to nursing homes. A village police officer that I knew remarked to my husband, "I thought Mary was a better nurse than to work there". Life in nursing homes has improved tremendously since that time. I believe this is due to better education and benefits for the caregivers as well as Federal and State monitoring and general awareness of family and friends.

Yet, my experiences have led me to believe there is an underlying depression in most elderly people, especially those confined to nursing homes. This may be due to loneliness and loss of mobility. In the quiet hours of the night, I have listened to many who shared with me their readiness to die. They are all alone and are tired of living and do not want to be burdensome to their families. Listening is the best form of communication and it is important for them to know we are there for them. I usually ask these patients if they believe in God and an afterlife and if they would like me to pray with them and for them. It is also important to let the physician know as a little medication may improve their disposition.

I worked in Long Term Care over the next twenty years. I worked as Night Supervisor, Staff Development Coordinator and Director of Nursing in different facilities. Over the years, I have heard some incredible tales of incidents that occurred. I will share some with you.

A colleague with little experience oriented a new nurse assistant on the night shift. The new NA was instructed to remove the residents' dentures at night, clean them and return them to the bedside for the next mornings use. The following night she collected all of the dentures in a basin and cleaned them as she was instructed. She never labeled to whom each denture belonged. How the basin of dentures got back to their individual owners remains a mystery.

On another occasion, a resident was sent to a hospital emergency room with discoloration of one foot and faint pedal pulses. In the ER, the discoloration disappeared when the foot was washed. Later, it was discovered that the woman had recently worn a new pair of shoes and the dye had ran causing the "discoloration".

As with any profession, maintaining a good sense of humor is required to keep things sane!

Over the years, I've worked closely with many nurse assistants who shared their eagerness to increase their knowledge. I became aware that the training available to them, though very advanced in the State of Illinois, left a lot to be desired. I decided to enroll in a "Train the Trainer" program offered by the Illinois Department of Public Health (IDPH). It was a week-long course provided to registered nurses to enable them to teach people interested in becoming Nurse Assistants and prepare them for certification.

In Illinois, the Certified Nurse Assistant course is 120 hours long (as of this writing). A minimum of 12 hours of Alzheimer's content must be taught in order to prepare students to care for patients with Alzheimer's disease.

The original course consisted of 80 hours of classroom where basic anatomy, physiology and practical skills such as bathing, dressing, taking vital signs, weights, intake and output measurements, transferring and repositioning.

The students were then assigned to patients in a skilled care setting. They provided direct care under the supervision of the trainer/instructor. When the course was completed, the students took an examination, and then took a skills test sponsored by IDPH. Upon passing, a student received a certificate of completion and was then ready to apply for a position as a Certified Nurse Assistant.

I attended the Rehabilitation Institute in Peoria, Illinois for certification in Rehabilitation Nursing. The Rehabilitation Certification course took four weeks. A nursing colleague and I travelled by car to Peoria where we stayed during the week. There were 12 students in the class from different parts of the state. The institute was affiliated with two Peoria hospitals where we did our hands-on clinical training. We were each assigned one patient.

We learned the basics of repositioning, transferring and range of motion exercises. We accompanied the patient to physical and occupational therapies and kept a journal on our patient's progress. It was amazing how well patients responded to therapy. They became encouraged as they regained mobility and strength. I completed the course by passing a qualifying examination. My dream was to share my knowledge with others someday.

That dream materialized when I was employed by Moraine Valley Community College in Palos Park, Illinois. I developed and taught a 40-hour course for R.N.'s on Rehabilitation Nursing Techniques. I also was involved with the teaching and training of new Certified Nurse Assistants.

I also had the opportunity to teach at Howe Developmental Center in Tinley Park, Illinois. Howe is a 1,000-bed long-term care facility for mentally disabled adults. A law passed in 1988 required mental health technicians employed there to become Certified Nurse Assistant's (CNAs) and I was contracted to provide the training.

Once again, I met some wonderful caring individuals and it was a pleasure to provide them with the additional knowledge and skills to obtain certification. Many of them had served in Vietnam and shared their experiences with me.

I want to share a poem written for me by one of my CNA students:

"Teacher: Usually unknown to you and
sometimes to ourselves.

You guide if not change our lives.

You have to be of a certain sort if not of
the same mold.

To give of yourself as you do to people
you hardly know.

I guess you could call it love,
not of a certain person but of all people.

For there is indifference among you
about what type of person sits behind the
desk.

Because you teach everyone as if they were
your own to the best of your ability.

Don't think you are not appreciated,
my teacher, because you are.

It may not be said out loud but I feel it in
my heart.

It is also proven by every student who passes your class.

That student is that much more prepared to become someone a little better than his forefathers.

A new generation, with a destiny to make this world a better place."

I encouraged my daughter and son-in-law to take the course for their own enrichment and as I watched them provide safe and gentle care to patients, during their clinical rotation, I knew my future was in good hands.

I thoroughly enjoyed teaching and trained many nurse assistants who continued in the nursing profession. I always attempted to instill a sense of respect, caring and hope for the patients assigned to their care. Over the years, I also learned much from my students.

IDPH mandated that skilled long-term care facilities either have a Director of Nursing with Rehabilitation Nursing Certification or utilize the services of a Rehabilitation Nurse Consultant on a part time basis. I provided consulting services to many long term care facilities in the Chicagoland area. My duties included, assessing new admissions for the appropriate restorative nursing program, assessing the progress of patients on current programs and providing in-service education to the nursing staff on restorative issues. Presently, Physical Therapists do these assessments and provide treatment.

I became a charter member of The National Gerentological Nurses Association (NGNA). They issued a quarterly magazine with numerous articles pertaining to diagnosis, treatment and care of patients with chronic illness and the realization that patients could live longer and healthier lives that are more meaningful. I attended the NGNA annual conventions offered in various states in the country. I met many nurses with similar interests in caring for the elderly and at the same time, I had the opportunity to visit many wonderful places in our beautiful country.

As time progressed, more equipment became available; Hoyer lifts, digital thermometers, mechanical scales, electric beds, to mention just a few. These advances have been a boon to nurses because it has saved time and has certainly prevented back injuries. Present day nurses accept this as normal, but for older nurses who started without them, they are truly miraculous. On one occasion, I asked a patient care technician (PCT) if she needed help weighing a patient. She told me the patient had a new bed with a scale. How awesome!

Modern technology has made the caregivers' lives easier but then again patients are living longer and can be more fragile and confused. It is certainly a challenge to reorient them and keep them safe. At one convention, I attended a seminar on Validation Theory. Validation is a practical communication method that helps reduce stress and enhance dignity in disoriented people. I have frequently used this in caring for confused patients. I have found that when patients are extremely confused it is easier for staff to agree with the patient than to try to reorient him, at that point. This prevents hostility or aggression from occurring.

While working as a staff nurse, I cared for an elderly confused patient named Mike who got out of bed at 2:00 a.m. and proceeded to get dressed. The CNA attempted to take his clothes away from him and put him back to bed. Mike became loud and hostile. He was attempting to strike the

CNA. When I intervened, I asked him where he wanted to go. He said he was going to a friend's funeral. I asked where the funeral parlor was and how he would get there. He named a funeral home on the Far South Side of Chicago and the bus route he would take to get there. He remembered the exact street names and bus numbers. I explained it was only 2:00 a.m. and the first bus left at 6:00 a.m., and it was cold waiting at the corner bus stop. I offered him some warm milk and told him that I would get him up in time for the bus. Mike drank his milk, got back into bed and slept soundly for the remainder of the night.

CHAPTER THIRTEEN

In the early 1990s, I had the opportunity to work for the United States Department of Health and Human Services (DHHS). The agency to which I was assigned was Healthcare Financing Administration (HCFA) but was later changed to Centers for Medicare and Medicaid (CMS).

I worked in this field as a Federal Surveyor for the next fourteen years. I was assigned to Region V, which encompassed the six Midwest states of Illinois, Indiana, Michigan, Minnesota, Wisconsin and Ohio. I did most of my survey work in Minnesota. Minnesota is a very beautiful state with many wonderful people. I even found a lake named Lake Mary. I have acquired some great friends in Minnesota. I did Long Term Care, Hospice and Home Health surveys as well as fraud, waste and abuse investigations.

To become a Federal Surveyor, one had to be a RN, have at least a B.S. degree and have some nursing experience, the more the better.

After orientation at the Region V Chicago office, I attended basic training in Baltimore, Maryland, which is the national headquarters for CMS. I had to pass a qualifying examination before I could conduct my first survey.

Healthcare facilities who wish to receive payment from the Medicare program require certification as complying with the Conditions of Participation (COP) set forth under Federal regulations. The certification is based on a survey conducted by a state agency on behalf of CMS. This agency is usually the State Department of Public Health.

Joint Commission is a private National accrediting organization that enforces standards that meet the Federal COP's. CMS has given authority to this organization to "deem" the healthcare facility in compliance with federal regulations.

Therefore, a facility that has received "deemed" status is usually not surveyed by State or Federal agencies. Surveys are never announced and facilities are expected to remain in compliance with the COP's. Occasionally, CMS surveyors conduct complaint investigations or validation surveys of facilities with "deemed status". Surveyors sometimes accompany Joint Commission for monitoring purposes. The Joint Commission provides CMS with any survey reports required of them.

Originally, we surveyed in groups of three or four depending on the size of the facility. Our observations and documentation had to be extremely thorough as the healthcare providers often challenged our findings. Later the survey process changed and we did "Federal Oversight and Support Survey" (FOSS) and occasional Comparative surveys.

I hope I haven't confused you with all the acronyms we used. When I first started working at CMS, it was like learning a new language!

The FOSS is when one CMS surveyor accompanies the State survey team and observes the survey. Each State agency conducts surveys of

Medicare certified facilities annually. The Comparative and FOSS surveys are conducted on a specific number of facilities based on the number of certified facilities in each state.

The fiscal year begins October 1st and ends September 30th. We often waited for the Federal budget approval before beginning our survey activity. This ensured that Health and Human Services could provide the money to CMS for survey expenditures.

The preparation for a survey was very detailed. After the offsite research of choosing the appropriate facility was completed, I then made travel arrangements including flight, car rental and hotel accommodations. Often, the facilities were located in small towns or rural areas and I had to travel long distances to find suitable hotel or motel accommodations. I often had a 7:00am flight from O'Hare to Ohio or Minnesota. Then, I picked up a car and drove 2 hours to an assigned facility. I worked 8 or 10 hours before checking into my hotel. The hours were often long, but the work was interesting, challenging and necessary.

The survey process involved observations, interviews and record review. A sample selection was based on the number of certified beds in the facility. I observed all aspects of patient care including wound care, foley catheter care, pressure sores, restorative procedures, positioning and transferring techniques and range of motion exercises.

Interviews consisted of meeting with administration, direct care staff, patients and families. I questioned staff on their knowledge of topics such as fire safety and abuse prevention. These interviews were an integral part of the survey, because we learned about the care patients were receiving.

The record reviews were long and tedious, but this was a vital component of the survey process. I reviewed patient charts, accident and incident reports, infection control protocols, pharmacy medication orders and written procedures for fire and safety protocols. Reviews of closed records helped determine if discharge planning and placement was appropriate.

An audit of employee records examined background checks, proof of citizenship and if employees satisfied annual in-service education requirements.

The facility survey included a tour of kitchen to determine if sanitation, food storage temperatures and appropriate menus for diet orders were in place.

The monitoring of laundry facilities was also important to ensure safe and appropriate handling of soiled and clean linens. Lastly, the entire facility was assessed for cleanliness and proper waste disposal. We checked that fire safety doors, alarms and exit lights were in working order.

I found the transition from "hands-on" nursing and teaching to being a Federal Regulator difficult at times. While observing a medication pass or a dressing change, I had to restrain myself from offering a helpful suggestion or discussing better techniques. I could not intervene unless injury to a patient was imminent and of course, that was never allowed to occur.

When the survey activities were complete, the survey team determined the findings and held an exit conference with the facility administration. The survey was far from over at that point! After travelling back to the Chicago office, our reports had to be entered into a database in a timely manner.

It was while working for DHHS that I first became acquainted with computers. Our survey reports and complaint investigations were computerized.

On one occasion, I did a Congressional report that had to be just perfect. After many hours of concentration and hard work, I began to print the lengthy report but nothing printed. I had forgotten to save it. Some angel of mercy, with more technical savvy than me, retrieved the document from the hard drive. After that, I learned my lesson. "Save early and often"

Once again, we worked as a team and supported each other in a discussion of findings and documentation procedures. A supervisor checked all reports and they often came back for correction and/or further explanation. Clarification was sometimes hard and I often thought to myself, "I was there, not the supervisor." Reports had to be based on observations and findings as they were often challenged in a court of law.

As I continued to gain experience in the survey process, I returned to Baltimore for additional training in Hospice, Home Health and Complaint Investigation protocols.

I did investigations of Federal Home and Community based waivers and interviewed both the recipients of the waiver program and those accountable for its distribution. I conducted congressional complaint investigations and completed data entry and report writing for all investigations and surveys. I was also involved in the training of new Federal and State surveyors. I met many wonderful people and saw excellent care given to our elderly and disabled people.

During the early days of my survey work, I frequently encountered patients who had restraints on. Restraints helped prevent confused elderly patients from wandering or falling. Many times multiple restraints were used, such as pelvic, vest and wrist. It was sad to watch elderly patients struggling to get free. Sometimes these patients were placed on large beanbags from which they could not escape. Now restraints are rarely used.

However, when a restraint is necessary, nursing staff removes them frequently so the patient can exercise and eat meals. Many awesome interventions are in place to keep people safe including getting a person out of bed, putting them into a wheelchair and bringing them to the nurse's station where they can be monitored. Frequent toileting and hydration help to decrease any anxiety the patient may be feeling.

I thoroughly enjoyed working as a Federal Surveyor. Federal Regulations are required to combat poor care and shortcuts. As a surveyor, I looked for the regulations not met; therefore, I looked for negative outcomes. I often felt I was unable to compliment the many excellent care-givers who worked in Rehabilitation and Long Term Care facilities. I must give credit to DHHS for the wonderful training I received while working there. Any training I was interested in was readily available.

At that time, I became certified in Gerontology and Legal Nurse Consulting. The work was always stimulating and worthwhile. During my time there, I also became computer literate and once again, the necessary training was always available.

One of my special assignments was in monitoring Illinois hospices for abuse of the Medicare Hospice Benefit. Another surveyor and I were assigned to this project, which was conducted over a period of many months. Again, hospices with a specific number of patients enrolled in the Medicare Hospice Benefit Program over a prolonged period of time were chosen. We received specific training on investigative techniques from the Office of the Inspector General (OIG).

Hospice is a concept of care for dying patients that involve the family. It is usually home based but there are some inpatient care facilities available for short-term and respite care. The movement started in the United Kingdom and I have been fortunate to visit the first hospice in London, which is St. Christopher's Hospice. I have also attended many lectures on Death and Dying presented by Dr. Eleanor Kuebler Ross who was a pioneer in the field in the United States.

Hospice surveys had to be meticulous and many hours were spent documenting our observations and interviews. It was imperative that our reports included specific person, place, time and occurrence, I often had concerns over these reports but the Federal Guidelines had to be followed and the benefit program protected from overuse and abuse.

Some recipients were babysitting their grandchildren on a daily basis, others were found gardening or shopping. Many patients were on the program for years, which was originally intended for short-term end of life assistance. Based on our findings, changes were made and the program is now tailored to prevent misuse.

During our investigations, we always received the utmost satisfaction from speaking with recipients and families about the care provided by hospice nurses.

During my observations as a Federal Surveyor, I saw wonderful interventions in caring for the elderly. One time I conducted a dining observation in a nursing home at noon. An elderly, well-dressed woman was seated alone at a small table by a window. As the dining room assistant delivered her tray, I saw the woman give her some money. I was concerned with the exchange of money.

The Director of Nursing informed me that when the resident came to live there, she refused to eat or leave her room, as she did not have money to pay for anything. One ingenious employee thought of play money. Now this woman pays for her care and tips generously. The next day I interviewed the resident who told me she was very happy and said that the food and services were reasonable. She even recommended I come to live there.

Throughout my years of surveying, I met some wonderful residents who shared many incredible stories of their earlier lives prior to coming to this country. I vividly remember two sisters, aged ninety and ninety-two respectively who were determined to teach me how to play cards.

On another occasion, I met a retired nurse who was over one hundred years old but extremely cognitive. When I asked her if she did her nursing with an oil lamp (as Florence Nightingale did), she laughed and responded "No, a little later". She shared stories with me of her home health work in the tenements in the New York waterfront district

One program I was extremely interested in LTC was restorative nursing. As people age, they need to maintain the activities of daily living as long as possible. On occasions when I have encouraged residents be more independent, I have had family members tell me" that is what YOU are there for". When I try to explain how important it is to move about and be as active as possible, some family members feel guilty and helpless to see a beloved parent ill. That is where encouragement and empathy are important.

When I surveyed, I always looked at the restorative programs available. It is incredibly sad to see old people lined up in wheelchairs staring into space for hours.

I was so proud to be a Federal Surveyor. I had come a long way from my first nursing adventure in Dublin, Ireland. I've had some wonderful experiences and I am always grateful to my parents for the sacrifices they made in providing the money for my nursing education.

Survey work involved long hours and much travel. Post 9/11, I often was tired of removing my shoes at airports, although I know that is necessary for our safety. I tried showing my Federal identification badge so I could pass quickly through the airport security but it did not work. I retired from DHHS but not from nursing.

CHAPTER FOURTEEN

My next position in the field of nursing was as a Legal Nurse Consultant for a medical malpractice law firm. The lawyer who interviewed me asked if I would have difficulty testifying against another nurse. I informed him that where negligence was involved, it would not be problematic but if I did not agree with the findings, I would readily tell him so.

During the cases I reviewed, I was horrified to see the lack of pertinent documentation provided by nurses. The old cliché "If it wasn't written it wasn't done" came to mind. I know in my heart that surely some nurse, on some shift, must have changed a wound dressing in a two-week period but the record failed to reflect that any dressing change had been done.

Falls and subsequent injuries are such frequent occurrences that a safety program is very necessary in health care facilities. Some examples of fall prevention includes not transferring a patient with left side weakness from the left side of the bed; and the patient who received sedatives or tranquilizers should be assessed for cognitive awareness and mobility prior to getting out of bed. Falls can be avoided.

Throughout my work for the law firm, I never found criminal negligence or the intent to do bodily harm, but I was saddened to see omissions in care and documentation that were grounds for a lawsuit.

I have continued to do part-time nursing in a skilled care unit. I really enjoy providing bedside care and I have learned through my own experiences that pain medication does not always work, I always return to access the patient's response and provide some additional support as needed.

I recently cared for a very old man with numerous aches and pain. He was angry that he had lost much of his independence. I tried to make him as comfortable as possible and in the morning, he thanked me for taking care of him. He told me I reminded him of his mother. When I asked him why, he replied, "She was very kind". I considered this a wonderful compliment.

When bedside medication verification was first introduced, I was very skeptical it would be time consuming and a nuisance. This is a system whereby each medication is scanned for the five "R's" - or Right's in administering medications.

- The Right Patient
- The Right Medication
- The Right Dose
- The Right Time
- The Right Route of Administration

A bar code is placed on the patient's identification band. Each patient's medication (generic name also) dose, time due, route appears on the computer screen. This process has certainly decreased medication errors. It is easy to review the medication administration record (MAR) in the computer to ensure that all medications have been administered timely. This is certainly a fantastic convenience for the nurse.

Over the years, I have travelled to many countries in Europe and Asia. I always inquire about what healthcare is available, especially for the elderly. I have seen long waiting periods for services and limited equipment.

A few years ago, my friend Sharon and I attended a convention in beautiful Scotland. Sharon's husband, Keith, was a lifesaver by driving us all around Scotland thus avoiding the double-decker buses. The topic of the convention was "Geropsych" which pertained to geriatric patients with psychological problems.

During two weeks of lectures, observations, and interviewing both caregivers and recipients, I found tremendous limitations in care. Social Services were more readily available than nursing care. One social worker explained that a disease state occurred when a person was "ill at ease" and if the social structure was intact people would not be ill. There was also cut off ages for the availability of some drugs and procedures.

One man told me when his wife turned sixty-five, Aricept (an expensive drug used for Alzheimer's) was no longer available for free and he could not afford to purchase it.

During our trip, Sharon and I also visited an "old age home". There was no evidence of any Restorative Care. People dozed in their chairs or just stared into space. It was suppertime and many caregivers stood over patients and spooned pureed food into their mouths. I commented on the use of finger foods, plate guards and specialized cutlery, which would enable the person to eat somewhat independently. I also recommended that the caregiver should sit while assisting the patient to eat. I told them about the Restorative Nursing techniques available in the United States.

The supervisor was very interested but did not have any available materials. When I returned home, I mailed her lots of information on Range of Motion exercises, transfer techniques, group exercises, and handouts that I had used when teaching Rehabilitation Nursing. Over the course of the convention I frequently told Sharon I was thankful to be an American Citizen and thankful for Medicare.

As I wind down my nursing career, my thoughts turn to the future of the nursing profession. With the advancement of technology, we have gained some and lost a lot as well. In some states there are trained medication aides passing medications instead of nurses. Physical therapy and occupational therapy personnel now do what nurses did in restorative and rehabilitation programs.

Hospitals are now businesses and our patients are our customers. We provide service not care. Heaven forbid if we ever mention we are short staffed. Staffing grids used to determine if adequate nursing staff is available reflect the number of patients a nurse gives care to but not the patient acuity level or the time it may take to care for each patient.

I cringe when I hear advertisements for various hospitals informing the public of their technology and success stories. I guess this is the age of technology. I see nurses dressed in scrubs, cords and sweats of various hues. However, whenever I visit my dentist's office, the dental hygienist looks so nice in a crisp white uniform. My granddaughter Madelaine tells me "Nana, you come from a different era". Perhaps I do.

I have interviewed many student nurses on their goals for the future. The majority of them have told me they want to earn advanced degrees and become nurse practitioners or nurse educators. I have asked about basic nursing and one student responded that would be a waste of her education. She said, "It doesn't take a nurse to give a bedpan". True enough, but how sad that it may be beneath us, to provide the most basic needs to our patients.

Bedside nursing care as I have experienced will change. There is a grave shortage of nurses and this will increase as older nurses retire. There is also a shortage of nurse educators for students interested in entering the profession. Perhaps trained technicians will provide bedside nursing needs.

CHAPTER FIFTEEN

Another area of change, which I have experienced over the years, is in Pain Management. This certainly has been beneficial to the bedside nurse as it is very frustrating to see a patient in pain.

Early in my nursing career, pain medication was prescribed sparingly. Analgesics were a scare commodity. Over the counter pain medication was very limited. I remember seeing a pain packet called "Aspro". It contained five pills and that was the only OTC pain medication available.

Narcotics such as Morphine or Demerol were ordered at 4 or 6 hour intervals and administered intramuscularly. If the pain was not relieved, nothing else was available until the time interval had elapsed. Nurses attempted repositioning, massage, cold compresses and prayer. Often, the pain medications were prescribed based on the patient's blood pressure. "Hold if Systolic BP is less than 90". When this order was in the chart, the pain medication was held if the BP was low.

In Europe, the advent of Hospice Care made pain relief a greater issue and better pain management evolved. Presently, pain is considered the fifth vital sign and patients are assessed for pain at frequent intervals. A pain scale has been developed and patients are asked to describe their pain on a scale from one to ten.

In my clinical experience, I have found that this is not always reliable. Some patients do not comprehend the meaning of the scale. I have seen patients who told me that their pain was a nine, while they were enjoying a program on T.V. I do know that some patients have a greater tolerance for pain than others do.

As with other technological advances hand held patented devices are now available to measure the skins response to pain. This device also monitors the effectiveness of the treatment option being used and can evaluate the degree of recovery following injury or surgery.

Pain medication is now prescribed more liberally. It may be given at 6 hour intervals around the clock and may have another analgesic prescribed for breakthrough pain. Patches of analgesic medication may be applied to the patient at 72 hour intervals. It is always important to monitor and document the patients' response to the prescribed pain medication. Therefore, the pain medication can be changed or the dose adjusted as the patient has the right to safe and adequate pain relief.

Post-operative pain is often treated with the use of a patient controlled analgesia pump (PCA). The pump contains pain medication as prescribed by the doctor. A syringe is connected to the patient's intravenous line. The pump can be set to deliver a small continuous flow of medication or an additional dose can be self-administered by pressing a button. The patient can control when they receive the pain medication and then the flow is not continuous. These pumps may also be used to control other types of pain. They have built-in safety features.

The total amount of analgesia a patient can receive is within a safe limit. The R.N. frequently checks the level of the medication as well as the patient's cognitive status and vital signs.

In the early 1990s, I became aware of a new therapy available to nurses to allow them to nurture and promote healing in patients, called "Healing Touch". The founder, Jean Montgen, R.N. introduced the program in 1989 as an in-service education program for nurses and it is now an International organization. Many universities, medical and nursing schools teach the Healing Touch program.

I decided to attend a weekend seminar. I learned that this is an energy-based approach to health and healing and utilizes patient biofeedback. Gentle touch stimulates the human energy system.

This is a non-invasive approach where the practitioner places their hands gently on or slightly above the body while the client is fully clothed. The patient and the client unite energetically to facilitate the client's healing. During the two-day seminar, I was the taught the technique and then practiced it on other students.

The session lasts 40-60 minutes. When I was on the recipient end of the therapy, I must say I experienced a relaxed and peaceful state both during and after the session.

Healing Touch can be used for any of the following:

- Pain Management
- Headaches
- Wound Healing
- Emotional Healing
- Stress Reduction
- Relaxation

At this time, Healing Touch is practiced in a variety of settings including Long Term Care facilities, Hospitals, Hospices and Private Practices. Medical insurance often covers the cost.

There is a cumulative effect of having multiple therapy sessions and naturally, the client and practitioner develop a stronger bond over time.

Back at the start of my nursing career, alternative therapies were unheard of. It is wonderful that treatments such as Healing Touch, Homeopathic

Medicine and Acupuncture are available and becoming more widely accepted as alternative or even complimentary methods of treating conditions.

CHAPTER SIXTEEN

As I reflect on my nursing career, I am profoundly grateful for the career options available to nurses at this time. When I began, a student nurse had only three choices. One could become a General Nurse working in a hospital setting, a Mental Health Nurse working in a Mental Hospital, or become a Nurse Midwife.

General Nurse training took three years with the option to specialize in either Mental Health or Nurse Midwifery with an additional year of training in the chosen field. One could omit the General Nurse training completely and spend two years working in the other two fields to become certified.

Today, nurses enjoy a wide-range of amazing career choices. There are Flight Nurses, Cruise Ship Nurses, Office or Clinic Nurses, Home Health Nurses, Hospice Nurses, Nurse Educators and Nurse Practitioner just to name a few. Nurses can represent Pharmaceutical, Insurance or Medical Supply companies.

There are many exciting specialties for a nurse to receive certification in. I've previously mentioned the areas in which I am certified: Legal Nurse Consulting, Gerontology and Rehabilitation. Certification is available for ER, Intensive Care and Pediatric Intensive Care just to name a few.

To become certified, one must study the subject thoroughly by attending classes and seminars or taking home study courses. Then one must pass the qualifying examination. The certification period is for two years, and re-certification requires a certain number of continuing education hours.

At the time I was certified, I was always on the lookout for seminars to attend. Now with the Internet, it is very easy to build up the required number of hours via online study options. I still attend some seminars, as nurses in Illinois are required to have 20 hours of continuing education to become re-licensed every two years.

With all these opportunities, and with the advancements in technology, it is easy to surmise that my robot friend on the back cover may one day have a place in nursing. I have read many articles recently on the use of robots in the future of nursing. I personally do not like the idea of cold metal hands.

Documentation is another big area of change for nurses. We wrote documentation by hand with few abbreviations allowed, and no luxury of "spell check!" At one time "PORK" Problem Oriented Record Keeping was the chosen documentation style. Then "SOAP" Subject, Object, Assessment and Plan became the way to go. It was sometimes challenging to describe or document essential areas of care under those guidelines.

Now we have computerized documentation software with appropriate check-off lists for medications, treatment and assessments. The appropriate headings are already in place and a nurse is unlikely to forget a required field. Episodical documentation can be included under nurses notes to describe a special occurrence or event pertaining to a patient.

I am now actively involved in Healthcare Information Technology and I often wonder how I managed the old way. I learned nursing informatics and the use of computerization for the administration and documentation of the medication pass. One of the greater benefits of computers in nursing care is the ability to retrieve data instantly. Information on laboratory values, x-ray reports, or vital signs are all readily available.

There were few male nurses in Europe in the 1950s. I once had a friend who fell in love with a male nurse and took him home to visit her family. When her father learned of his career choice, he refused to allow them to marry. The male nurse eventually joined the police department, they married, and as far as I know, they lived happily ever after.

We have come a long way since then. Over the years, I have worked with many excellent male nurses and during my own hospitalization, some male nurses cared for me.

I now provide care in another dimension. I am a Minister of Care in my church. I visit the sick in nursing homes and in their own homes. I bring Holy Communion, pray with and listen to them.

As I reflect back on my years as a nurse, I feel so privileged to have experienced and learned so much. I also feel honored to have provided care to so many. Many years ago, I read an acronym for CARE:

C = Courtesy
A = Attitude
R = Respect
E = Encouragement.

I have always tried to provide those to my patients

As I complete this narrative, I have one major concern. That is the tremendous waste of resources. It upsets me to open a patient's bedside drawer and find it cluttered with three rolls of adhesive tape, two dressing packs, four toothbrushes, three bottles of soap and two sticks of deodorant, etc. As our population ages and requires more care, resources will be less available. Now is the time to prepare for this.

I believe part of the orientation for every new healthcare employee should include a section on cost containment. Employees should be reminded frequently of the need to conserve supplies. Perhaps my concern stems from the earlier days of my career when we often had to make do with less by way of supplies and technology. In order to treat our patients successfully, we frequently had to improvise.

I still remember an old Irish poem I learned as a child.

> "Willful waste makes woeful want
> And you might live to say
> I wish I had the crumb of bread
> That once I threw away."

I will conclude with a prayer for nurses I received from a student many years ago and which I still say daily:

Give to my heart, Lord, compassion and understanding.

Give to my hands skill and tenderness.

Give to my ears the ability to listen.

Give to my lips words of comfort.

Give to me, Lord, strength for this selfless service

And enable me to give hope to those I serve.

Amen.

Glossary

Accu-chek	A brand of blood glucose testing devices manufactured by Roche Diagnostics.
Acetone	A liquid found in extremely small amounts in normal urine, but larger quantities occur in the urine and blood of people with diabetes.
Albumin	A type of simple protein, widely distributed throughout the tissues and fluids of the body.
Autoclave	A machine that sterilizes instruments or materials with high pressure and heat or pressurized steam.
Banshee	A female spirit in Irish mythology, usually seen as an omen of death.
Big Ben	The large bell that chimes the hours in the clock tower of the Houses of Parliament in London
bronchiectasis	Chronic dilation of the airways to and within the lungs, causing coughing and excessive mucus production
Bucks traction	An apparatus for applying skin traction on the leg in which adhesive tape is connected to the skin and to a suspended weight.
Bunsen burner	A portable tube-shaped gas burner with an adjustable hole to control air intake and flame type, used in laboratories
cephalic presentation	Head first position
cerebrovascular accident	This general term encompasses such problems as stroke and cerebral hemorrhage.

cervical traction	Traction of the neck
Circle-electric bed	A bed used for spinal cord injured patients
craniotomy	Cutting open the skull to expose the brain, especially for brain surgery
enema	The insertion of a liquid into the bowels via the rectum as a treatment, especially for constipation, or as an aid to diagnosis
episiotomies	An incision sometimes made to enlarge the vaginal opening in the late stages of labor to prevent tearing and facilitate the birth
Fowlers position	An inclined position obtained by raising the head of the bed about 60 to 90 cm to promote better dependent drainage after an abdominal operation.
Friars Balsam	A complex mixture of natural medicaments including benzoin, storax, balsam of Peru, balsam of Tolu, aloe, myrrh, angelica and alcohol. Also called also balsam traumatic.
gas gangrene	A form of gangrene, caused by aerobic clostridia bacteria, in which gas forms in injured body tissue
great omentum	Peritoneal fold suspended from the greater curvature of the stomach and attached to the anterior surface of the transverse colon.
hemodynamic monitoring	Monitoring of the physical aspects of the blood circulation.
HIPAA	Health Insurance Portability and Accountability Act
Hoyer lift	A patient lifting device
hurling match	An Irish field sport resembling hockey and lacrosse that is played with broad sticks and a leather ball that is passed from player to player through the air
(HBOT) hyperbaric oxygen treatments	A pressurized chamber that allows for the delivery of oxygen in higher concentrations for therapeutic benefit

hypertonic saline solution	A salt solution, sufficiently concentrated to cause osmotic shrinkage of cells immersed in it.
inhalation treatment	A treatment delivered by breathing in medication or moisture into the lungs
Kardex	A system for tracking care and medications
ketone	Ketones are substances that are made when the body breaks down fat for energy. Ketone test checks for ketones in your blood or urine.
laparotomy	Surgical incision into the abdominal cavity through the loin or flank
lateral position	Side lying
liniment	A liquid rubbed into the skin to relieve aches or pain, e.g. one containing alcohol and camphor
lorry	A large truck designed to carry heavy loads; usually without sides
magnesium sulfate enemas	Type of enema used to reduce intracranial pressure
Matron	Matron is the job title of a very senior nurse in several countries, including the United Kingdom and the Republic of Ireland although the title Clinical Nurse Manager is used.
myocardial infarction	Heart attack
papyraceus fetus	A fetus in a multiple pregnancy, which has died in vanishing twin syndrome. Due to mechanical compression in the womb, the result resembles a flattened, parchment-like paper attached to the placenta.
pedal pulse	A pulse felt at the top of the foot
PEG tube	A feeding tube, percutaneous endoscopic gastrostomy (PEG).
perineum	The area between the thighs extending from the coccyx to the pubis and lying below the pelvic diaphragm.
post partum depression	A common depression occurring after giving birth
postural drainage	A treatment that helps drain mucus from the lungs.

poultices	A hot, soft, moist mass, as of flour, herbs, mustard, etc., sometimes spread on cloth, applied to a sore or inflamed part of the body
prone position	The body when lying face downward
recumbent position	A reclined position
Rhesus factor	An antigen present in the red blood cells of 85% of humans. A person with Rh factor is Rh positive (Rh+); a person without it is Rh negative (Rh-)
Russell traction	Splint less type of balanced lower limb traction affected by holding the skin of the whole leg with adhesive plaster.
semi-recumbent position	Reclining position at 45 degrees
sister	A senior female nurse
specific gravity	The ratio of the mass of a solid or liquid to the mass of an equal volume of distilled water at 4°C (39°F)
sphygmomanometer	A device to take blood pressure
Stryker frame	A frame used to immobilize spinal cord injured patient
supine position	Lying face upward.
Swanz-Ganz catheter	The passing of a thin tube (catheter) into the right side of the heart.
Tincture	An alcoholic or hydroalcoholic solution prepared from vegetable materials or chemical substances. iodine tincture
Tincture of Benzoin	Provides skin protection and acts as an antiseptic prior to the application of adhesives or skin barriers.
titrated	A method to determine the concentration of a solution
Trendelenburg position	Head lower than the feet position
ward sister	Nurse

About The Author

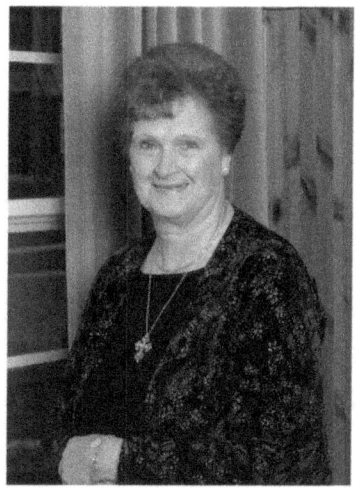

Mary lives in Bridgeview, Illinois. She enjoys reading, knitting, crocheting and baking. She loves visiting with family and friends. She returns to Ireland frequently to visit family and friends there. Mary also enjoys the ocean, especially from the deck of a Princess cruise ship.

www.ingramcontent.com/pod-product-compliance
Lightning Source LLC
Chambersburg PA
CBHW051527170526
45165CB00002B/641